The Alpha Plan:

Healthy Eating in College and Beyond

* * *

Mariam Manoukian, MD, PhD

With Kim Fielding

"So, what's it like in the real world? Well, the food is better, but beyond that, I don't recommend it."

Bill Watterson

Preface

The goal of this book is to make you love healthy and nutritious foods, the type of food most people hold preconceived notions about. "I eat only foods that I like." You should still say that. It is going to take some experimentation and time to find foods you like that are also healthy and don't promote disease.

The reality is, you can never force anyone to eat what he or she does not consider tasty, even if it is considered very healthy. Maybe once, but that is it. You need to try a variety of healthy foods to find the ones you like. You could make a trip to a local health-food store to help you find some new food choices and presentations. You could also try our recipes. They are quick, inexpensive, and tasty enough to be prepared over and over. Once you develop a taste for nutritious foods, fast food will lose its appeal and seem disgusting in comparison. By age 40, many look back with regret on the health decisions they made in their lives. With this book, you can avoid that, and our mission will have been accomplished.

* * *

Acknowledgements

We would like to thank our families for their unfailing support and love. A special thanks to Elize Manoukian, for her meticulous and talented editing at every stage of the book, Dr. Jerry Manoukian and Robert Maximoff, for their masterful editorial comments, Sona Arabian for her digital art work used for the cover page, and Nathan Fielding, for creating the name "The Alpha Plan."

I would like to thank my colleagues and friends Drs. John Bilezikian, Jane Lombard and Patrick Kearns for their extensive review and valuable comments.

* * *

Table of Contents

Introduction

With regard to food choices, today some colleges provide better food than others. However, in general, students are left to fend for themselves; they are for the first time the decision makers. What to put on the plate, what to shop for, and what to eat or not eat is solely up to the student.

The "Freshman 15" is an expression that refers to the weight that many students gain in their first year of college. The causes of this phenomenon seem to be common sense for some, but others struggle to understand why they so adeptly pack on the pounds. Notable causes are:

- Not understanding the importance of healthy eating
- Stress and comfort eating
- Eating late at night
- Keeping unhealthy snacks nearby
- Unlimited sugary drinks
- Lack of exercise
- Eating unhealthy cafeteria food
- Drinking excessive amounts of alcohol
- Emphasis on low-cost, "economical" foods that are usually refined carbohydrates and low-quality fats.

Proper eating is a safety issue. College is also the place where most learn the effects of excessive drinking and its ugly consequences. Often, college food is the first independent eating for most young adults. And eating right sets you on a healthy life trajectory. Moreover, poor eating habits impact mental health. If ignored, the Freshman 15 slowly progresses and, by age 40, advances to 60 excess pounds. And that is when all the troubles really start; diabetes, high blood pressure, high cholesterol, achy joints, sleep apnea, and many other diseases creep into a person's everyday life.

For college students, health is not a priority, because illness is not a reality. "Treat your clothes from new and your health from youth," says a popular Russian proverb. You're given one body and it's not replaceable. Love it and take care of it! College is the time to realize that and start taking care of your health, before it's too late.

Beating the Freshman 15 means eating healthy and staying fit while having a very busy schedule. It's hard to find time to exercise and easy to grab fast food. But even after college, things do not become any slower, and it's always going to be easier to live an unhealthy lifestyle. It is important to develop the healthy habits earlier in life even though they might be more time consuming.

Many say "you are what you eat." I say "tell me what you eat and I can tell you who you are." It's that easy. This book is your tool to transform Western living and its destructive consequences into healthy living that will keep your mind and soul healthy in college and thereafter.

Mariam Manoukian, MD

* * *

The Alpha Plan for Collegiate Life and Beyond

"The way to get started is to quit talking and begin doing."

Walt Disney

Let's be realistic—it's easy to gain weight and hard to lose it. It is easy to know what to do but very difficult to do it. In college you have a major advantage compared to people over forty. Your metabolism is perky and weight loss is simpler than it is later in life, although it is still difficult. Nowadays, everyone has a relative with diabetes and is aware that most people with diabetes have to watch what they eat to keep their blood sugars from skyrocketing. All of us should know that if we watch what we eat, most of us will never develop diabetes, heart disease, or cancer.

Health should be treated in the old-fashioned style, by embracing preindustrial principles and rejecting modern food processes that encourage obesity. Since the post-Depression and postwar rationing days, cheap and abundant foods have become a staple of Western culture and economy. Cost-effective methods of eating were introduced with good intentions. As a result, previously unknown substances penetrated our food, endowing it with an eternal shelf-life, bright color, incredible sweetness, and palatable flavors. Then came the glamorous commercials.

Did you know that obesity has surpassed the diseases caused by cigarettes or excess alcohol? About 70% of Americans are overweight and obesity is the fastest-growing disease in the developing world. More people die from obesity and its complications than from cancer. Not everyone is ready for weight loss or needs to lose weight, but everyone will benefit from learning and implementing a healthy lifestyle. We called it an Alpha Plan. It is a novel American lifestyle that arms you with tools for healthy living, improving your well-being, helping you lose or maintain weight, and cutting the risk of developing diabetes, heart disease, or cancer in the future.

The Alpha Plan is your blueprint for college health and beyond. Alpha, the letter beginning the Greek alphabet, symbolizes going back to the beginning. This book is not a weight loss guide but can help you along the way.

The book is divided into four parts. The first two parts are dedicated to topics that shed light on healthy living and teach simple and effective ways to improve the college lifestyle. Each chapter enlightens you on a useful concept in nutrition, physical activity, and environmental factors affecting health and suggests an action point.

Part 3 and part 4 are all about foods, cooking, menus, and simple recipes that are can-do and affordable for a student budget. They are about certain foods that you can make when you don't have access to a stove and a variety of meals and recipes for the times when you already have a stove in your apartment. It is about healthy eating at the cafeteria, on-campus dining out, and snacks for late-night cram sessions.

Part 1.
All you need to know about health

1. Why do people gain weight?

While the weight gain of college students is very similar to that of other age groups, there is an advantage in your favor. Young people are able to burn calories faster. That is known as faster or more robust metabolism. Following are the causes of weight gain typical for all age groups:

Genes—Thanks, Mom and Dad.

Age—At least you're getting wiser! However, age is not an important element for college students, unless you stay in college for a decade.

Alcohol consumption—Now that you're in college, you're (legally) old enough to consume to your heart's content. The forbidden fruit of alcohol—besides its brain-clogging effect—carries heavy calories and frequently is the sole reason for college weight gain.

Food abundance—Almost every change in diet for the last 40 years has increased food portions and made it easier for the consumer to eat calorie-dense food.

Stress—When God closes a door, we open a box of cookies.

Environment—There is too much food around us.

Immobility—Your grandmother was more active than you are. She had no car and no Wikipedia.

Genes are strands of DNA that we are given whether we wanted them or not. Blue eyes, the grey strand of hair at age 26—these factors are set in your genes. Vascular and metabolic diseases are passed on the same way. Until DNA-altering surgeries are developed, there isn't a whole lot that we can do about them, except for learning. By improving your habits, you can prevent the inevitable.

Knowing about your parents' medical conditions can be very useful. If your parent had a heart attack at the age of 50 or younger, then you want to find the rest of your risk factors for heart disease and prevent or treat them. If your parent has Type 2 diabetes, then the best way to prevent it happening to you would be losing weight and keeping it off.

The concept of the "thrifty gene" has been well elucidated and proven. Our remote predecessors starved and ate only when there was food. As a result, they developed a strong trait of accumulating their energy for the days when their prey eluded them. But for us, the "days" have evolved into the only four hours from lunch to dinner. Thanks to our hunter-ancestors, we have been programmed not to let go of the weight and the food that we encounter.

Alcohol consumption in inexperienced college students is a known cause for injuries, death, sex abuse, drunk driving, vandalism, and many other nasty consequences. Weight packing seems benign in comparison with those effects, but weight gain that starts with alcohol abuse in college can be the beginning of a lifelong battle with alcoholism and weight problems. Alcohol isn't directly stored as fat, so a "beer belly" will most likely develop over time. Eventually, drinking interferes with your general lifestyle and messes up the appetite. Drinkers are known to eat more and usually the worst types of foods. Exercise often becomes a lower priority. Remember, just because you can drink doesn't mean you always should.

Food abundance has one of the greatest impacts upon the waistline, something that should not come as a surprise. Everyone knows that we eat more than we should, so the simple solution is to eat high-nutrient, low-calorie foods, and limit the amount you eat. Unfortunately, almost everything advertised on TV is low-nutrient, high-calorie food. The food industry revolution supersized, enlarged, processed, fattened, colored, sweetened, and salted many foods with the sole purpose of selling more of them to you. The industry invented coupons, 99-cent burgers, free refills, bonus fortune cookies, and complimentary candies by the front counter—all of these and many others are conventional baits. These processes successfully made their way to the tables of naïve consumers. Remember, everyone, unfortunately even your relatives, is trying to make you fat. You're your sole advocate in keeping your waistline. And this book is your advocate, too.

Stress creates multiple mechanisms that induce weight gain. Healthy people get sick and sick people get sicker when faced with emotional trauma. Chronic stress is associated with elevated cortisone production, which promotes a rise of glucose and weight increase in the abdominal area. That is a physiological response, but there is nothing physiologic about stress. Stress wears down the body and makes people feel sorry for themselves and pamper themselves with denial. The stressed mind looks for comfort food—sugary and fatty.

Immobility has become an integral part of Western society since the Industrial Revolution, as we looked for new and inventive ways to simplify life. Television, computers, remotes and video games are indelible marks of our reality. If poor diet is one head of the obesity dragon, then a sedentary lifestyle is the other one.

* * *

2. How much should you weigh?

There are dozens ways of finding out how much you should weigh, but the truth of the matter is that your ideal weight is unique and should not be based on a comparison to others or based solely on numbers. Most tables take into consideration your height, and some have your frame and gender plugged into the equation, but none takes into consideration your age, genetics, activity level, ethnicity, number of pregnancies, and other details contributing to weight.

Most students do not start as overweight in college. If you weren't overweight when you started college, then your ideal weight for the rest of your life shouldn't increase more than 20 pounds. If you start underweight, then it's a good idea to gain some weight.

Besides looking into the mirror, there are multiple graphs and tables that will tell you the truth. The most commonly used measurements to evaluate weight are the Body Mass Index (BMI) and Waist Circumference (WC). Your BMI is your weight in kilograms divided by the square of your height in meters. BMI = weight (kg)/height (m^2). Note that kg = 2.2xlb and 1 meter = 39.37 inches.

Obesity is defined as having a BMI over 30 kg/m^2. A BMI exceeding 25 kg/m^2 is considered to be overweight. If your BMI is more than 25, then it's time to learn why and what can you do about that. The ideal BMI for women is approximately 19–23 kg/m^2 and is 20–24 kg /m^2 for men. If you are a larger frame person, then up to 25 kg/m^2 is okay. However, if your BMI is less than 18kg/m^2, then you need to make sure that you eat enough calories. Aiming for a BMI of 17 is an unhealthy and unsafe goal. Be realistic and honest with yourself. It is crucial to be comfortable with your weight and concentrate on living a healthy life.

Waist circumference is another measurement for weight. It is measured by placing a tape measure around your bare abdomen— just above your hip bones—and bringing it together on your belly button. Be sure that the tape is snug, does not compress your skin, and is parallel to the floor. Relax, exhale, and measure your waist. Women with a waist measurement of more than 35 inches or men with a waist measurement of more than 40 inches are considered overweight, but in college you're better off another 3 inches less.

As a matter of fact, WC correlates with medical diseases more than weight or BMI. Thinness doesn't correlate with health. Somehow we started to compare the types of weight gain to fruits: apples when people gain the weight around their stomach and pears when the weight concentrates more around the thighs. The apple type is also called the android or masculine type, because men will gain the weight more in that pattern. If you've seen women in paintings of Peter Paul Rubens, then you know what a pear shape, gynoid, or feminine weight gain is. Pear shape is considered to be a metabolically healthier weight gain. Most people who gain their weight around their stomachs become candidates for metabolic syndrome, a condition that predisposes the person to the development of diabetes and heart disease. If your BMI is above normal, it might be because you exercise a lot and have an eight-pack. Arnold Schwarzenegger probably has an elevated BMI, but he certainly doesn't have any fruit shape. However if your waist circumference is larger than 32 for a girl or 37 for a boy, then you absolutely need to work to bring your weight down, and that will bring you waist circumference down. This is a BMI chart to help you figure out where you stand.

* * *

Find Your Body Mass Index (BMI)

Height (inches)

Weight (lbs.)	58	59	60	61	62	63	64	65	66	67	68	69	70	71	72	73	74	75	76
100	21	20	20	19	18	18	17	17	16	16	15	15	14	14	14	13	13	12	12
105	22	21	21	20	19	19	18	17	17	16	16	16	15	15	14	14	13	13	13
110	23	22	21	21	20	19	19	18	18	17	17	16	16	15	15	15	14	14	13
115	24	23	22	22	21	20	20	19	19	18	17	17	17	16	16	15	15	14	14
120	25	24	23	23	22	21	21	20	19	19	18	18	17	17	16	16	15	15	15
125	26	25	24	24	23	22	21	21	20	20	19	18	18	17	17	16	16	16	15
130	27	26	25	25	24	23	22	22	21	20	20	19	19	18	18	17	17	16	16
135	28	27	26	26	25	24	23	22	22	21	21	20	19	19	18	18	17	17	16
140	29	28	27	26	26	25	24	23	23	22	21	21	20	20	19	18	18	17	17
145	30	29	28	27	27	26	25	24	23	23	22	21	21	20	20	19	19	18	18
150	31	30	29	28	27	27	26	25	24	23	23	22	22	21	20	20	19	19	18
155	32	31	30	29	28	27	27	26	25	24	24	23	22	22	21	20	20	19	19
160	33	32	31	30	29	28	27	27	26	25	24	24	23	22	22	21	21	20	19
165	34	33	32	31	30	29	28	27	27	26	25	24	24	23	22	22	21	21	20
170	35	34	33	32	31	30	29	28	27	27	26	25	24	24	23	22	22	21	21
175	36	35	34	33	32	31	30	29	28	27	27	26	25	24	24	23	22	22	21
180	37	36	35	34	33	32	31	30	29	28	27	27	26	25	24	24	23	22	22
185	39	37	36	35	34	33	32	31	30	29	28	27	27	26	25	24	24	23	23
190	40	38	37	36	35	34	33	32	31	30	29	28	27	26	26	25	24	24	23
195	41	39	38	37	36	35	33	32	31	31	30	29	28	27	26	26	25	24	24
200	42	40	39	38	37	35	34	33	32	31	30	30	29	28	27	26	26	25	24
205	43	41	40	39	37	36	35	34	33	32	31	30	29	29	28	27	26	26	25
210	44	42	41	40	38	37	36	35	34	33	32	31	30	29	28	28	27	26	26
215	45	43	42	41	39	38	37	36	35	34	33	32	31	30	29	28	28	27	26
220	46	44	43	42	40	39	38	37	36	34	33	32	32	31	30	29	28	27	27
225	47	45	44	43	41	40	39	37	36	35	34	33	32	31	31	30	29	28	27
230	48	46	45	43	42	41	39	38	37	36	35	34	33	32	31	30	30	29	28
235	49	47	46	44	43	42	40	39	38	37	36	35	34	33	32	31	30	29	29

3. What the hell am I eating?

All food contains three main nutrients and sources of energy: carbo-hydrates, protein, and fat. On top of that, food has water, minerals, and vitamins. With enough knowledge and observation, you should be able to distinguish the prevalent nutrient in everything you eat.

Nature has given us a variety of produce, but most of what we buy in the supermarket is man-made. Natural foods like meat, fish, milk, and eggs are combinations of fat and protein. Whole grains, legumes, and vegetables contain carbohydrates and protein. Nuts are unique natural foods that contain all three nutrients, but mostly fat. All of these foods are found in nature and are usually sold along the perim-eter of the supermarket. Around the fringes of the store are foods made by minimum processing, like fermenting and culturing. This in-cludes yogurt, cheese, tofu, and other dairy and soy products. The rest of the food is partially or completely made by food manufacturers.

When food passes through our digestive system, it is broken down into nutrients that can be used for a variety of purposes. Proteins break down to amino acids, fats to free fatty acids, and carbohydrates to simple sugars, sugars being the prime source of energy. The left-overs are deposited into the liver and muscles; the remaining energy is stored as fat. The human body has multiple areas of need for fats, such as hormones, cell membranes, nerve sheaths, and padding.

We use protein for its structural value: it is used to make hair, cell membranes, antibodies (our immune system), and enzymes. Of course proteins, fats, and carbohydrates are needed by the body. The important question is, how much of each?

Each of the nutrients produces different amounts of calories. Protein and carbohydrates contain 4 calories per gram, while fats contain 9 calories per gram. Obviously, fats are more calorie dense and, in excess, easily become contributors to obesity.

Protein is a structural building block for our bodies. Those building blocks include a unique chemical structure called amino acids. There are many kinds of amino acids, 20 of which serve as building blocks for making proteins. Eight of these amino acids are called "essential amino acids." Our bodies cannot manufacture them and we need to get them from food to survive.

We refer to any protein containing all eight of these essential amino acids as a "complete" protein. Animal products (meat, fish, dairy products, shellfish, etc.) contain all of these eight essential amino acids.

Plant-based proteins are typically missing one or more of these eight essential amino acids, like a Scrabble set that is missing one or more letters. The trick to using plant-based proteins, as we will see, is to combine different plant groups (such as beans and grains) to achieve a complete protein.

Protein from animal sources is mixed with water, fat, and cholesterol. Protein from vegetable sources comes mixed with fiber and varying amounts of carbohydrates (in beans, lentils, mushrooms) or fat (in nuts and seeds). Cholesterol is only found in animal-based products, as is vitamin B12. Whole grains contain protein, but, once refined, bleached, or polished, they lose much of it.

* * *

4. Satiety and protein

From a weight-control perspective, protein is proven to give a feeling of satiety or fullness. The sense of satiety is likely secondary to the release of intestinal hormones in response to protein intake. These peptides directly affect the satiety center in the brain and make us stop eating. An adequate protein intake also means you are eating less fat and carbohydrates, increasing muscle mass.

The typical daily requirement for protein usually varies from 0.6–1.0 gram per kilogram of body weight, depending on age or health condition. Failing to balance protein is a potential cause of health problems. Too little protein would halt growth and healing, while too much protein is hard on the digestive tract and kidneys. Excess protein can also cause calcium loss from bones. If a protein comes from meat and contains saturated fats, then the excess translates to a hardening of the arteries.

Typically, it is recommended that we obtain 12%–20% of our daily caloric intake from protein. The typical caloric intake for an adult should be about 1,200–2,000 calories, which comes to 45–75 grams of protein daily. Three ounces of lean pork, fish, or chicken, or one can of sardines, contain roughly about 20 grams of protein. One cup of milk contains 8 grams of protein, whole-grain cereal contains 5 grams, and ½ cup of nuts about 10 grams. In addition, there are many plant foods with a protein content rivaling meat. These include nuts, seeds, soy products, and beans. Thus, a handful of (shelled) sunflower or pumpkin seeds can easily contain 5 to 10 grams of protein. A soy hot dog can easily contain 9 grams of protein. Tofu contains twice the protein ounce for ounce as egg white.

Nuts and seeds are great additions to daily meals. They can be added to the salads, cereal and breads. They contain fats, which happen to be unsaturated, and can improve the cholesterol, in contrast to the saturated fats found in meat. Two ounces of walnuts contain 14 grams of protein, mostly from omega-3s, though they also have 340 calories.

* * *

5. Know your fats: Not all fats are bad for you

For the last 40 years, since fats have been shown to increase heart disease and cancer, fats have been under relentless attack from nutritional scientists and the food industry. But are all fats equally harmful?

Actually, fat is an important nutrient. We need fat to produce hormones, to absorb certain vitamins (A, D, E, and K) from the intestines, to give us energy (at 9 calories per gram), and to keep us warm in the winter.

Fat and oil are basically the same thing, except oil is liquid and fat is solid at room temperature. There are five basic types of fat:

Saturated fats are usually solid at room temperature. The major sources of saturated fats are butter, lard, ghee, meats, dairy, and coconut oil. Margarine also contains significant levels of saturated fats, but is to be condemned for other reasons. This type of fat should be eaten in moderation, so ease up on the Big Macs, which have 10 grams of saturated fat. You're better off with coconut oil, which has been shown to improve the health of your hair, skin, and waistline.

Cholesterol is a fat we are all familiar with, either from your parents' medicine cabinets or commercials for breakfast cereals. However, there is also cholesterol in food, which has a minimal impact on the cholesterol levels in our blood. Cholesterol is found in foods such as egg yolks and also in a variety of foods in conjunction with saturated fats.

Trans fats are the worst fats and are unknown in nature. These are created in a lab under high temperatures, by reintroduction of hydrogen atoms into fatty acid chains, causing double bonds to randomly convert into single bonds. This process is called hydrogenation, and many foods on the market contain hydrogenated or partially hydrogenated fats. Vegetable shortening is another name for these fats. These fats contain trans-fatty acids. We can't use them the way we usually use fats (to build cell membranes, nerve coatings, and hormones). They are one of the major culprits of weight gain. They raise the bad cholesterol and lower the good cholesterol.

These partially hydrogenated fats give foods the properties of long shelf life. If you buy pastries made with these compounds and accidentally lose them in the back of your cupboard, you will note that they still appear fresh months and years later. Processed foods—margarine, snack foods, french fries, doughnuts, and cheap baked goods—are primary sources of trans fats. Previously thought to be harmless (in the 1980s margarine was considered "better" than butter), these trans fats are shown to harden the arteries and have other harmful effects (like suppression of immunity) on the body.

A direct correlation has been shown between consumed hydrogenated fat and body fat. On a scale from −10 (bad) to 1 (good), trans fats score −10, saturated fats score −5, polyunsaturated fats score 1, and omega-3 fatty acids are +5. In 2005 the U.S. government, in its dietary guidelines to Americans, recommended keeping trans-fat consumption as low as possible. Based on this information, health officials started to come up with laws to ban trans fats. The American Heart Association (AHA) in 2006 recommended keeping trans-fat consumption under 2–2.5 grams per day. Just to enlighten you, an order of McDonald's french fries without anything else contains 8 grams of trans fats. Now, all food packaging is required to show the food's trans-fat amount, so the consumer (who actually pays attention) can actually see if there are trans fats or not. "Zero trans fats" on labels is quite popular these days. Interestingly enough, it doesn't necessarily mean that there are no trans fats at all; it actually means that the food has, at most, 0.5 grams of trans fats per serving. That is still very good. For the last couple of years, many areas like New York, Philadelphia, and others banned the use of trans fats in restaurants. This year California is joining the others in watching the drama of fast-food companies "making their food taste good without trans fats."

Now it is time to praise fats. Eating very low fat has been shown to have a less beneficial impact on health than eating foods full of good fats. The verdict of the fat story is: Don't try to eliminate fats completely, because they are important. Use olive oil as your preferred oil.

Monounsaturated fats are healthy for the heart and cholesterol levels. Monounsaturated fatty acids, or MUFA, are the main constituents of olive oil. Canola oil, peanut oil, and certain nuts like walnuts and pecans also contain preferentially monounsaturated fats. It is well known that, traditionally, people consuming a Mediterranean diet rich in olive oil have lower rates of heart disease.

Polyunsaturated fats are found in vegetable oils, canola oil, flax oil, peanut butter, almond butter, and fish oil. As it turns out, unsaturated fats tend to be associated with lower cholesterol when compared with saturated fats. These can be omega-3, omega-6, omega-9, and others. Both omega-3 and omega-6 are essential fatty acids, so our body doesn't make them and we should get those from food. With the evolution of the Western diet, we started to get more omega-6s than omega-3s in our diet. The next chapter discusses how to increase the consumption of omega-3 fatty acids.

* * *

6. Omega-3 fatty acids are essential

The omega-3 fatty acids, along with omega-6 fatty acids, are called *essential*. Essential means that our body needs them for health, and because we cannot make them, we need them in our diet. For the last 40 years, with the changes in eating habits and the formation of the typical Western diet, the ratio of omega-3s to omega-6s went from 1:3 to 1:10, or in some cases 1:20 or 1:30. It happened because our consumption of processed and prepared foods increased dramatically, bringing down our natural and whole-food consumption. Omega-3 fatty acids have anti-inflammatory properties, whereas omega-6 fatty acids tend to promote inflammation. Vegetable oils, such as corn, peanut, sunflower oil, and margarine are examples of omega-6 fatty acids. Overconsumption of omega-6s in people who consume enough omega-3s negates the positive effects of omega-3s. The Western diet is shown to provide only 15%–20% of these essential nutrients.

The omega-3 fatty acids which are important in human nutrition are α-linolenic acid (ALA), eicosapentaenoic acid (EPA), and docosahexaenoic acid (DHA).

DHA and EPA are two omega-3 fatty acids found in fish and fish oil. In major studies, EPA is shown to improve all causes of mortality, trimming cardiovascular risk and improving triglycerides, blood pressure, and heart rate. DHA is required in high levels in the brain and retina as a physiologically essential nutrient to provide for optimal neuronal functioning (learning ability, mental development) and visual acuity in young and old alike.

Since 2000, daily intake of 300 milligrams of DHA has been recommended to all pregnant women because it helps the growth of the fetal brain.

Tuna, sardines, mackerel, and herring are also DHA-rich species. It is hard to eat fish every day, but one to three servings a week is not hard to do at all. As you've probably heard, there can be problems with eating fish. Farm-raised fish may contain antibiotics or other toxins. Fish farming can be harmful to the coastal environment. Wild-caught fish may contain mercury. Fish that typically contain high levels of mercury are shark, swordfish, and mackerel, whereas shrimp, canned light tuna, salmon, and catfish are generally thought to have low levels of mercury.

Take omega-3 fatty acids seriously. Their health benefits are widespread and the danger is virtually nil.

Omega-3 fatty acids can also be obtained from plants. ALA is another kind of omega-3 fatty acid and is found in flaxseed oil, dark green leafy vegetables, and canola oil, as well as nuts, such as walnuts, and beans, including soybeans. When included in the diet, flax oil or crushed flaxseeds exhibit multiple beneficial effects, including improvement of cholesterol profile and anti-inflammatory processes, as well as improved work of the digestive system.

Another oil to consider is hemp seed oil, which contains large amounts of omega-6 and omega-3 fatty acids in a ratio (3:1) that is useful to our bodies. It can be considered perfect oil and is currently widely available in healthy supermarkets. Canola and vegetable oils also contain some omega-3 fatty acids, but in less favorable proportions of essential and other unsaturated fatty acids. Sources for omega-3s differ, but here are some general examples:

3 ounces of pickled herring = 1.2 grams of omega-3 fatty acids
3 ounces of salmon = 1.3 grams of omega-3 fatty acids
3 ounces of halibut = 1.0 grams of omega-3 fatty acids
3 ounces of mackerel = 1.6 grams of omega-3 fatty acids
1½ teaspoons of flaxseeds = 3 grams of omega-3 fatty acids

Fifteen grams (1 tablespoon) of flaxseed oil provides 8 grams of ALA, which is converted in the body to EPA and then DHA at an efficiency of 2%–15%, and 2%–5% respectively.

Eggs produced by chickens fed a diet of greens and insects produce higher levels of omega-3 fatty acids (mostly ALA) than chickens fed corn or soybeans. Walnuts are one of the few nuts that contain appreciable omega-3 fat, with an approximately 1:4 ratio of omega-3 to omega-6. Acai palm fruit also contains omega-3 fatty acids.

* * *

7. What do you need to know about carbs?

Carbohydrates, or carbs, are extremely important for our body functions. They are the perfect source of energy needed for daily life—breathing, eating, digesting—and also for exercise. Carbs are easily taken up by the muscles and liver, which store glycogen that gets used when needed. Vitamins and minerals tend to appear in foods rich in carbohydrates.

Just like fats, there are different types of carbohydrates. There are simple carbohydrates, complex carbohydrates or starches, and fiber. Simple carbs are single or two-sugar molecules. We get simple carbs from sugar, corn syrup, and high fructose corn syrup, which are found in candy, juices, fruits, sodas, and just about any other product in the supermarket. These taste sweet, are easy to absorb, and momentarily increase the blood sugar. Increased blood sugar triggers an insulin surge that brings the sugar down, but also increases the fat storage. Bringing the blood sugar down quickly makes the person crave more sugar.

The complex carbohydrates include starchy foods. The main sources of starch include breads, rice, pasta, any grains, potatoes, and cereal. The body breaks down starch into simple sugars as it is absorbed from the intestine. Just like simple sugars, complex carbs raise the sugar level in the blood, but not as fast.

Fiber is a carbohydrate that is not digested but helps food move in the gut, lowers cholesterol, and slows down the absorption of other carbs.

The amount of insulin secreted by the pancreas depends on the amount and type of carbohydrate in the meal, and is affected by the rate at which the carbohydrate is absorbed. The popular Atkins diet restricts carbohydrates to very small amounts, contradicting the guidelines of the American Heart Association and American Diabetes Association. Too much carbohydrate restriction is an extreme measure, but some carbohydrate restriction and understanding is important for successful weight management.

* * *

8. What do you need to know about the glycemic index?

The glycemic index (GI) is a numerical index that ranks carbohydrates based on their rate of raising the sugar in the blood stream. Why is it even important for you to know the GI of the foods you eat? Because you want to stay away from foods that are high in GI.

GI uses a scale of 0 to 100, with higher values given to foods that cause the most rapid rise in blood sugar. The lower the GI index, the better the carbohydrate that you eat. Pure glucose serves as a reference point and is given a GI of 100. Glucose ranks as 100; white bread, candy, and fruit juices also rank close to 100. Carrots, apples, pears, plums, mushrooms, root vegetables, broccoli, zucchini cabbage wheat bran, barley, oats, grainy breads made with whole seeds, yams, lentils, kidney beans, and garbanzo beans are low glycemic index foods. Low GI foods are digested more slowly and cause less insulin to be released. There is good data that slowly absorbed, low glycemic index foods are associated with increased HDL (good cholesterol), help people lose weight, improve insulin sensitivity, and reduce the risk of diabetes. As an analogy for the glycemic index, imagine an accounting department at a factory. If the money trickles in slowly throughout the year, one accountant might be able to keep all the books. If all the money for the year comes in over a few days or weeks, then a larger team of accountants will be needed. The pancreas needs to secrete a lot more insulin in response to a sudden load of sugar in the bloodstream. As a result of increased insulin secretion in response to high glycemic foods, a person eventually develops insulin resistance, weight gain and if the person has genetic predisposition he or she is at high risk of developing diabetes.

* * *

9. Portion control

Portions and calories are often interrelated. The bigger the portions are, the more calories are being consumed, and the more the calories are being consumed, the more body fat is being accumulated. If we had to classify the culprits in the epidemic of obesity in this country, then increased portion sizes would likely win a gold or at least a silver medal. Since 1980 there has been a steady increase in portion sizes served at restaurants. The way restaurants competed against each other was by luring customers through portion sizes and prices. People were seduced by adds for *oversized* and another decade later by *supersized* servings. Words like "big," "extra," "grande," "tall," "whopper" attract the stressed mind. The sizes for servings of soft drinks went from 8 ounces to 16, to 24, and finally to 32 ounces. Each increase doubled the sugar count and brought the calorie count up almost by 100 or more. But it's not just that. Twenty years ago, one hamburger was about 330 calories. Today the same hamburger is 590 calories. Two slices of pizza were 500 calories and today there are 850 calories. A large popcorn at a movie theater used to be 270 calories; today it's 630 calories.

There was another trick to the marketing wizardry—the price for the next larger portion of food is minimally different from the previous portion. The marketing math is seducing—you pay only 30% more but get a 100% larger portion.

In a recently published study that compared different types of diets (low carb vs. low fat), it was shown that portion control was the parameter that correlated the most with weight loss. How do we decrease portions to the level of 1980?

* * *

10. Exercise and physical activity

The terms "physical activity" and "exercise" are often used interchangeably but really are not synonymous. Physical activity encompasses any movement that involves muscle contraction and leads to an expenditure of energy. Exercise is a subcategory of physical activity, and that is where going to the gym, running, and jogging come in. These examples are structured, deliberate, and repetitive movements designed to improve or maintain some component of physical fitness. Exercise is the more arduous cardiorespiratory and strength training, whereas physical activity can actually include washing dishes, walking up a flight of stairs, and standing while talking on the phone instead of sitting. All of these involve the muscles and engage the metabolism.

Students who run or go to the gym daily have already mastered a healthy exercise pattern and, as a rule, don't need to fight their weight unless they have extremely poor eating habits. Teenagers and young adults have a metabolic advantage over their middle-aged counterparts. But although their metabolism is higher, burning consumed calories is very difficult. To work off the calories from 2 ounces of potato chips, you need to run 3 miles in 30 minutes.

Studies have shown that the amount of exercise is just as important as the intensity of it. Walking is the healthiest form of exercise, and if you're walking about an hour a day—the total amount it takes to walk between classes—that is adequate. If you find yourself not even walking that much, make the extra effort for the sake of your metabolism. Short bouts of intense exercise can prevent fat accumulation in the liver and improve the metabolism.

To find out how many steps you take per day, use a pedometer. A cheap pedometer can be purchased online for less than five dollars. Use it for one day to calculate the steps used in your basic daily routine and whether this is a good amount. Ten thousand steps per day and 70,000 steps per week is a healthy average. While these numbers seem ridiculously high, they can be easily achieved by walking instead of driving, or choosing the stairs over an escalator. If you totally miss this goal, don't be discouraged! Work a trip to the farmer's market, a hike, or even a quick jump-rope session into your busy schedule.

Physical fitness is actually more than exercise. It is a general state of good health, usually as a result of exercise and nutrition. Fitness is achieved through healthy eating and exercise. But how much and what kind of exercise does it take to be considered fit?

Not long ago the American Heart Association recommended 30 minutes of exercise five times weekly. In 2005 the recommendation changed to 210 minutes per week, and a more recent recommendation is higher than that. More than 210 minutes per week helped people to lose weight and maintain the lost weight.

Some important facts about fitness: it is associated with better immunity, better neutrophil (cells that fight infection) action, less inflammation, less depression, less atherosclerosis (hardening of the arteries), less mortality, better HDL (good) cholesterol, less LDL (bad) cholesterol, better diabetes control, better sleep, and more productivity.

Aerobic exercise training is an effective way of achieving these goals. Most exercise we do, like walking, jogging, biking, dancing, yoga, Pilates, swimming, etc., is aerobic. *Resistance training* also induces beneficial changes in insulin sensitivity, glucose storage, and muscle mass. Most YMCAs will offer such classes. Consider taking a body-building class. Keep walking, park your car far from your destination, take stairs, do a morning jump rope, use the exercise bike. Even when you feel tired, make an effort to achieve fitness—it will pay off.

* * *

11. Hormones and appetite

Over time, biological science has discovered more culprits involved in obesity. There are several known hormones that impact our appetite, and many more are probably still unknown . Three of those are anorexigenic, which means that they are supposed to lower the appetite or cause anorexia. The hypothalamus is the area in the brain where the centers of appetite regulation are situated.

Insulin is secreted by the pancreas in response to the intake of food that contains glucose. Rising insulin levels affect the hypothalamus and cause a reduction in food intake. Unfortunately, this feedback is lost in type 2 diabetics. When a person develops insulin resistance, the feedback breaks down. Insulin resistance is a term describing the pancreas, producing more insulin than normal to control the blood sugar in response to carbohydrate consumption. Many insulin resistant people will develop diabetes during their lifetime.

Leptin is a hormone secreted by our own fat cells in response to food consumption. When it goes up, it signals satiety, or a feeling of being full, in the hypothalamus, which tells the body it is time to spend energy, kicking up the metabolism. In other words, leptin is signaling to the brain that it is time to stop eating and start spending the calories. Overweight people have a glitch in this otherwise well-designed system. It's called leptin resistance. Some people are genetically leptin deficient, and they get very obese very early in their lives. But for most people it's not genetic (or may be genetic but not confirmed) and there is no leptin deficiency. With prolonged overeating of nutrients that are high in fat and high in carbohydrates, people develop leptin resistance or factual leptin deficiency.

Peptide YY is produced by the small and large intestines and inhibits the appetite. This peptide is a most potent appetite suppressant, and there is a field of investigation for use as a possible appetite suppressant drug.

Ghrelin is produced by the stomach and signals hunger and a desire to eat. Just like with insulin resistance in obesity, ghrelin becomes confused, and even when people are overfed, ghrelin levels are decreased. Interestingly, obese people have low ghrelin levels and high leptin levels. Anorexia nervosa, on the other hand, is associated with high ghrelin levels following negative energy balance. Hormones are confusing.

The best way to avoid this vicious circle is to stay a normal weight. The best time to do it? In college. Why not earlier? Because college is when you are finally the decision maker. If you are already overweight, here is the good news. Now, more than any other time, your metabolism is good, and it's much easier to burn calories and lose weight.

* * *

12. Be aware of food guidelines

In the last 30 years, since obesity started to be recognized as an actual disease that can initiate a slew of other deadly diseases, the U.S. Food and Drug Administration, the American Heart Association, American Diabetes Association, and many other associations in the food sciences have flooded the public with guidelines that pointed the confused and naïve consumer in different directions. It turned out that what was thought to be bad for us wasn't so bad, and what was advertised as good for us was even worse than the bad things.

"Saturated fat is bad" was the slogan of the 1970s and '80s and, as a result, *partially hydrogenated fats*—representatives of polyunsaturated fats—were unfortunately created. The *low-fat* label was claimed to be better, and the *nonfat* movement should've saved the world. To give an example, that was when whipped cream and coffee creamer were made with cornstarch. As a result of national recommendations for a low-fat, carbohydrate-based diet, fat intake decreased by 5% in men and 9% in women, and daily carbohydrate intake increased by 168 calories in men and 335 calories in women. That is not so surprising, as women are known to have more of a sweet tooth than men. A corresponding increase in obesity occurred in both genders. In 1971, 45% of men were overweight, but in 2001, 70% were overweight. Among women, the numbers were 41 % in 1971 vs. 62 % in 2001. Unfortunately, national dietary guidelines to some degree are implicated in the national obesity epidemic. Advertising by the food industry has taken dietary guidelines its own way—as a new way to make more profits. "No cholesterol, no fat" is written even on soft drinks. It is required by law! "It doesn't have fat or cholesterol; it has to be good for me," concludes the naïve consumer. Duh! If it had any fat in it, then it would be soup, not soda. It is important to follow the contemporary science and recommendations but stay away from food fashions. For now, ignore the foods that are called "low fat" or "no fat." Those labels are for dumb consumers. Most of those foods will have sugar or high fructose corn syrup as their first ingredient, and that *will* make you fat!

In 2005 the U.S. Department of Agriculture changed the food pyramid into a more personalized version, with a little person climbing the stairs on the pyramid, thereby emphasizing the role of physical activity. In 2011 the "new" pyramid was abandoned and the USDA adopted a new symbol for healthy eating, a colorful plate that emphasizes whole grains; eating more green vegetables, fruits, and legumes; avoiding fruit juices; and eating lean meats and low-fat dairy products.

A lot of thought was put into that (choosemyplate.gov). It is certainly easier to understand and healthier than the previous pyramids. Science is catching up with social demand and guidelines are changing, but eating whole foods (those that aren't processed or refined) instead of whatever is in the plastic bag with nutritional gibberish is always going to be guideline to follow.

* * *

13. What is the best diet?

Fad diets are either based on food fashions or created by marketing experts. In the 1990s and early 21st century, a new discovery was made. Dr. Atkins came up with the idea that carbohydrates are our real enemy, not fat, and the public jumped from one extreme to the other—low-carb bread and low-carb pasta flooded the market. There were many other diets as well—McDougall's (low fat, starch based), Ornish's (very low fat), South Beach diet (low carb, less fat, high glycemic index) and most recently the Dukan diet (rich in lean protein, with a restricted food list and four steps to follow.)

The exclusion diets taught us something very important—eating low fat or low carbohydrate as a permanent lifestyle is sometimes unhealthy and almost impossible to follow. Yes, the meats should be lean and never fried, the desserts should go back to birthday parties only, fatty dips and margarine should go to hell, but, please, enjoy your omelet, lamb chop, free-range chicken, fish, plain yogurt, nuts, and seeds. Dr. Atkins and his followers recommend a low carb diet, and right then they threw the baby out with the bathwater. The phrase "low carbohydrate" makes little sense unless you specify what type of carbohydrate. Yes, you should avoid simple carbohydrates and refined sugars, sodas, juices, candy, sweet desserts, and white-flour products, but, please, enjoy the kind of carbs that you find in vegetables and fibrous fruits, legumes, and whole grains. Many successes of low-carb diets are explained because simple sugars are cut out of the diet, but if the person continues to eat large amount of whole grains and fruits, that might hinder the weight loss.

When the popular exclusion diets were compared, both diets had a large number of dropouts (people who didn't stick with the program), and the ones who stayed in for a year had similar amounts of weight loss. That is not surprising. Any time you exclude certain foods you cut down on calories, but the low-fat diets are hard to maintain, and the low-carb diets can promote certain cancers and atherosclerosis.

On low-carbohydrate diets, people eat not only too much fat but also too much protein, creating an extra strain on the kidneys. Low-carb diets bring in a high phosphate load and foods that are flooded with antibiotics, pesticides, and hormone residues that are harmful.

Meats, cheese, tofu, eggs, dairy, nuts, whole grains, and legumes are great sources of protein and should be regulars in your diet, but not overeaten.

The best diet is simply based on two important principles: the type of food and amount of food. Whole foods, plants, fruits, lean meats, high fiber, and whole grains are the types of foods you need to eat. Eating normal portions and avoiding seconds, as well as "big," "large," and "grande" sizes for whatever you're eating, is the second principle. These two principles form the foundation of the Alpha Plan or Alpha Diet, but it is also about eating at least three times a day in a relaxing environment. It is about reading labels and avoiding simple carbohydrates, high fructose corn syrup, partially hydrogenated fats, food coloring, and artificial sweeteners. It's about learning to cook and creat new dishes and colorful meals. It's a diet that will be totally recognized and appreciated by your grandma or great-grandma and will not shock her.

* * *

14. Alcohol and weight

When we talk about alcohol, the old movie called *The Good, the Bad, and the Ugly* comes to mind. Alcohol tolerance and consumption are influenced by the person's genetics, gender, the type of drink, and, most importantly, the amount of alcohol being consumed by the person. Moderation is the key word, but, for many people, moderation is the hardest thing to do, particularly in college.

The legal drinking age varies around the world. Some cultures allow drinking from a young age; some prohibit it completely. Like Indonesia and the United Arab Emirates, the United States has set the drinking age at 21, although many start before or after this age.

There are ample statistics about illegal use of alcohol in colleges, and quite prominently in fraternities and sororities. Thirty-one percent of college students met criteria for a diagnosis of alcohol abuse and six percent for a diagnosis of alcohol dependence, according to questionnaire-based self-reports about their drinking. Drinking goes through stages from moderate to excessive, and from funny and relaxed to dangerous and life-threatening. Alcoholics typically cannot drink one or two beers or a glass or two of wine. It's all or none, and that is the "ugly." Alcoholism doesn't obey common sense, just like any other type of addiction. It is an illness that is difficult to treat. For many students it is the forbidden fruit if they haven't reached the age of 21. For most it's a control issue. Some alcoholics, luckily, go into permanent remission. Those are the ones who can't drink alcohol at all, or the "ugly" happens again.

The "bad" in alcohol has a different face. It is more common, and this is what hinders weight loss. These people are functional; they just drink too much. They don't end up in the emergency rooms but are suffering from many effects of excessive alcohol consumption. One of those is the effect on their weight. Interestingly, alcohol, despite its calories that are higher than carbohydrates, does not turn into fat. What excess alcohol does is stop the usage of fat as a fuel, because alcohol (or, more precisely, acetate) is now used as a fuel. Just like excess carbohydrates (except that carbs also can easily turn into fat), the fat stores are preserved and weight loss is hindered. When alcohol is consumed in large amounts, people are at risk for obesity, sleep apnea, breast cancer, depression, and insomnia, as well as arrests for DUI and homicide.

With regard to weight loss, alcohol is shown to increase the appetite. Alcohol is also known to decrease the level of testosterone in men and women, and as a result more fat is stored and muscle turns into fat.

But what is a large amount anyway? It's quite simple - more than 1 drink per day for women or more than 2 drinks per day for men. Others consider alcoholism in women who drink more than 14 drinks per week and men who drink more than 21 drinks per week. One drink is the equivalent of 12 ounces of beer, 5 ounces of wine, or 1.5 ounces of hard spirits.

Here are some tips how to avoid the "ugly" and the "bad" in alcohol.

* Make right decisions for yourself.
* Always eat before drinking.
* Keep track of how many drinks you have.
* Drink water along with alcohol—one glass after the first drink, two glasses after the second.
* Keep an eye on a friend who drinks too much.

There are some good things about moderate alcohol consumption. Nothing about weight loss, but people who consume small amounts of alcohol daily are shown to have a lower incidence of diabetes, heart attacks, strokes, dementia, and even arthritis.

* * *

15. Gender difference in regards to weight gain

Boys and girls and men and women take being overweight differently. Women and girls want to be thinner than they are. They constantly try to lose weight and frequently are upset about their weight. Men, on the other hand, are less neurotic about their weight and lose weight more easily once on a diet. Not fair. Men usually have more robust metabolism than women of the same age. Women have more body fat, have more hormone influences, are more emotional, and tend to try new, fashionable diets more than men. Comfort food is more typical for women. But women are also more knowledgeable in the basics of nutrition. Men are less likely to read labels or follow a diet, and are lucky to have more muscle mass that gives them a more active metabolism, even as they age. There is something about the Y chromosome that makes them less anxious about their body image and naturally resistant to try diets. However, as a result of the male's calm attitude, there are more obese boys than girls, and the difference is getting bigger.

A healthy woman of normal weight has a body fat content of 25%, while a healthy man of normal weight has a body fat content of 15%. It is all about hormones. Fat percentage also goes up with age. In observational studies, the average weight gain in college freshman was 5.04 pounds for males and 5.49 pounds for females. Weight gain was more related to increased alcohol consumption in men and increased workload in women. Women are typically more stress-eaters and increased pressure promotes that kind of eating. Studies have also shown that African American young women are at an even higher risk of weight gain than white women of the same age.

* * *

16. Effect of cigarettes and pot on weight

In two distinctly different ways, smoking pot helps you gain weight. Cannabis triggers an increase in appetite, which is why one of its best-known medical uses is in patients with anorexia and HIV/AIDS. Getting the "munchies" is the desire to eat sweet and fatty foods. Pot also gives the sense of bliss, so the person cares less about his or her appearance as well as the weight. For regular smokers, life becomes comforting in any shape. People who smoke pot on a regular basis, otherwise known as stoners, invariably gain weight. Studies have been done and have not shown any change in metabolism as a result of smoking pot. There are no calories in marijuana, and it's not the pot itself but the increase in food intake that causes the weight gain. A national survey demonstrated that marijuana use was higher among students who participate in other high-risk behaviors, such as binge drinking, cigarette smoking, and having multiple sexual partners, and among students who perceive parties as important and religion and community service as not important. Partying and binge drinking are well-known contributors of weight gain.

Tobacco, on the other hand, is known to prevent weight gain and causes some increase in metabolism from nicotine. Cigarette smokers also suffer from a chronic bad taste in their mouth that decreases the appetite. Obviously smoking is not any better than excess weight, so that should not be used to counteract the weight. Smoking and obesity are equally evil, not a good way to fight one with the other.

Heavy smokers sometimes gain weight after they quit. The appetite is better and the metabolism is slower. The more cigarettes a person smokes, the more weight the person can potentially gain after they quit. The weight gain is due to the fact that the person is looking for something to help cope with anxiety; this is otherwise known as "oral gratification." That "something" to put in the mouth after quitting smoking is food. Chewing gum can help. Having healthy snacks like celery or carrot sticks around also helps. Some programs also recommend toothpicks or a straw or mints. But the best way to overcome the weight gain after quitting smoking is taking up a new, healthy habit, such as walking, exercising, cooking, or yoga.

* * *

17. Obesity and sex

Sexual dysfunction is not brought up as a result of obesity as often as diabetes and heart disease, but that doesn't make it any smaller an elephant in the room. A person's sexual life is affected by his or her physical weight, hormones, and emotions at any age, and all three of those are interrelated. Excess weight creates poor body image and decreased sexual desire, which goes right back and makes the person comfort himself or herself with food. If not faced and worked on, the issue gets worse and weight grows. Sexual intercourse is awkward and the enjoyment is less, and this is well correlated with the amount of excess weight. The physical restrictions placed on the obese person by his or her weight often make sexual activity too difficult or strenuous. In addition, a constant lack of energy and feeling of lethargy will tend to reduce the desire for sex. Another impact obesity has on sexuality is a psychological one. Obesity brings along with it lowered self-esteem and often feelings of shame. These feelings lead to an unwillingness to display the body or make oneself vulnerable to one's partner.

Men in some cultures find a women with curves attractive, and the term "love handles" has been used to describe a plentiful, sexual body. But hardly any man or woman can find a morbidly obese person in an apple shape attractive, and that hurts many. The way a person gains weight is purely genetic. Body image and self-esteem both go down the drain with rising BMI.

In a study by Binks from Durham, half of the obese people (BMI above 41) had no sexual desire. In normal weight population, this percentage is around 2%.

Hormones like testosterone, the major libido hormone, go down in those who are overweight. It has been shown that BMI is inversely proportional to testosterone levels. In fact, when testosterone goes down, weight loss becomes harder, because the famous Y-chromosome-related fast metabolism shuts off.

Here is the good news: Weight loss by itself can completely fix the problem. Making changes in lifestyle has a positive emotional impact, allowing obese persons to feel some level of control over their situation. Sexual satisfaction is a basic human need, and it's just one more key reason to care for your health.

* * *

18. The aftermath of the holidays

Most everything about the holidays is about food. Sure, there are lots of family gatherings, parties with old and new acquaintances, skiing, fireplaces, flights and airports, lots of laundry, and stress, but mostly holidays are about food. As a result, statistics show that most Americans gain weight during the holidays: somewhere from 0.4 to 5 pounds. Interestingly, overweight adults tend to gain more weight than people with normal weight.

Most people don't have the willpower to resist the temptation of familiar tastes. Sweet, sour, greasy, crunchy, chocolaty, minty, alcohol: we serve our common temptations and then can't stop eating. Cold weather doesn't help. People crave sugary foods when they are cold. What can be better than a cup of hot chocolate with marshmallows? Not sleeping enough and feeling tired also stimulates the appetite for calorie-dense foods. Snacking on nuts, seeds, dried fruit, and dark chocolate seems like a healthy thing to do, but those also are full of calories. The worst part is the guilt feeling and the remorse. Socializing for the sake of socialization without overeating and drinking is not easy but is possible. After having some appetizers, walk around with a bottle of water, or have sparkling water in a large wine glass. And maybe it's too late to say this—but the only way to stop after one cookie is to avoid that first cookie. A tangerine is the best way to finish a meal. Just perfect sweetness.

* * *

19. Zits and food

What you put in your mouth affects your body, your mind, and your skin. But it's not just that simple. Plenty of people eat horridly but still have okay skin, and many young girls abstain totally from sugar and don't notice too much improvement of their skin. Many factors affect the skin—genetics, hormones, stress, and food.

Acne or a zit is a clogged pore that gets inflamed. Sebaceous glands produce more oil, and skin bacteria feast on it, causing inflammation. Just about anything that increases inflammation will promote acne.

Stress is certainly a big factor—it increases the inflammation. Chronic stress causes elevated production of cortisol, adrenalin, and androgen from the adrenals. All of these hormones make the skin oily and inflamed. Teenagers have oilier hair and skin, and they are the largest consumers of anti-acne medications. As you might've noticed, not many grandparents show up with zits. They are stressed, all right, but do not get acne. They pretty much lack hormones (testosterone goes down and estrogen pretty much disappears). So maybe the biggest contributors to acne are hormones. Not that simple! Every teenager has plenty of hormones but not everyone gets heavily hit by acne. If your parents had acne in their younger years, then expect the same propensity from your own skin.

Now about food: the foods that create inflammation are the same foods that create diabetes and heart disease: fried foods, fast food, packaged foods, sugary foods, and foods full of trans fats. Imagine what the effect of the greasy pizza is—your whole body gets oiled in saturated fats, and so does your skin. Raw vegetables, berries, green tea, whole grains, fish, and fish oil are all anti-inflammatory foods. The so-called inflammatory foods are the creation of food industry and are famous for lacking any natural vitamins and microelements. Nine out of ten teens do not eat enough vegetables. I'm sure the face of that one teen looks fabulous.

You can add vitamins supplements, but it's never the same. There are many players involved in acne formation—you have control only over your food. Eating raw, colorful, seasonal vegetables is the best for the skin. Calming down will help, too, but you can't change your hormones and genetics.

* * *

20. High fructose corn syrup: the bittersweet saga

Once upon a time, food chemists manipulated corn syrup by changing the glucose in sugar to fructose, creating an inexpensive sweetener that wormed its way into the majority of foods in supermarkets. Like so many other advances in technology and food processing, high fructose corn syrup (HFCS) turned into one of the most tangible causes of obesity.

Until the 1970s, most of the sugar we ate came from sucrose, which was derived from sugar beets or sugar cane. Sucrose, otherwise known as table sugar, consists of equal amounts glucose and fructose. Fructose is sweeter than glucose and even small increase of its percentage will increase the sweetness. While most of the world continues to eat mostly sugar, in the United States, sugar from corn (corn syrup, fructose, dextrose, dextrin, and especially HFCS) gained popularity as a sweetener because it was much less expensive to produce.

HFCS is composed of 55% fructose, instead of 50% fructose, as is found in fruits or honey. In fruit, the ratio is usually 50% glucose and 50% fructose. Fruit contains fiber, which slows down the metabolism of fructose and other sugars, but the fructose in HFCS is absorbed very quickly. Most commercial fruit juices have HFCS added to emphasize sweetness.

In 1980, the average person consumed 39 pounds of fructose and 84 pounds of sucrose. In 2004, the average person ate 83 pounds of fructose and 66 pounds sucrose. Because HFCS is so cheap, it can be added to almost anything imaginable—bread, pastries, cookies, candy, juices, sodas, jams, peanut butter, yogurt, ice cream, chocolate, condiments, canned soups, ad infinitum. Basically, HFCS is ubiquitous in processed foods. If you ignore the fine print of ingredients, you almost certainly will consume it many times per day.

In the past, fructose was considered beneficial to people suffering from diabetes, because it causes only a modest rise in blood sugar. However, research on other hormonal factors suggests that fructose actually promotes disease more readily than glucose. A recent study published by the journal *Cancer Research* directly linked fructose consumption to triggering pancreatic cancer cells, and potentially other types of cancerous cells, to grow more quickly. And because fructose can only be metabolized by the liver, it has been shown that teenagers consuming HFCS suffer from early fatty liver, a condition that was previously unheard of in young people.

Fructose requires less insulin because it acts like fat. It then clogs liver cells, therefore increasing insulin resistance in the liver and creating a prediabetic condition. This "free" fructose interferes with the heart's use of key minerals like magnesium, copper, and chromium. In addition, HFCS has been implicated in elevated blood cholesterol levels, particularly high triglycerides, formation of blood clots, hypertension, gout, and cardiovascular disease.

Peter Havel, a nutrition researcher at the University of California, Davis, who studies the metabolic effects of fructose, has also shown that fructose fails to increase the production of leptin, a hormone produced by the body's fat cells which promotes satiety. This mechanism is extremely convenient for fast-food restaurants purveying supersized options. If you are eating or drinking something that doesn't suppress your appetite center (such as a soda or a burger bun) then you can "enjoy" bigger and bigger portions. Therein lies the conspiratorial genius of HFCS.

One 12-ounce can of soda has as much as 13 teaspoons of sugar in the form of high fructose corn syrup. A 20-ounce soda has about 20 teaspoons of HFCS. No wonder that in 2000, it was shown that the average American consumes 31 teaspoons of HFCS daily. Today, more than 10%–15% of our daily energy intake in the typical U.S. diet comes from fructose; less than 20% of that comes from fruits.

The data on the negative effects of HFCS is overwhelming. This is not favorable, of course, to the manufacturers of HFCS, the Corn Refiners Association. This organization launched a major ad campaign in 2010 to retaliate against the bad press and convince consumers that HFCS isn't the evil it has been made out to be. This is evidenced by the association's cheesy and trite commercials, usually featuring concerned loved ones "exposing" the goodness of HFCS and then sharing some in the form of popsicles or juice. Do not be fooled by the evil corporation in sheep's clothing. Its motives are as rotten as the teeth of a consumer who doesn't pay attention to his or her high fructose corn syrup intake.

* * *

21. The first three letters in "diet" spell...

We've all been in this situation: you're ordering a meal that's heavy on calories, so if you get a diet drink, it cancels out, right? Wrong. Just because diet drinks are calorie free doesn't mean that they are risk free. Zero calories can seem good, but artificial sweeteners are bad for you. So what, exactly, is the matter with them?

1. Most artificial sweeteners (AS) are chemically made and not found in nature.
2. AS were introduced within the last 40 years, meaning your grandmother didn't eat them.
3. There is scientific evidence that AS cause diabetes, metabolic syndrome, and obesity as much as sugar (possibly more).
4. AS confuse the brain by providing sweetness without calories, leading to a subconscious connection between the two.

There are four main sweeteners that we see or use on a daily basis. This chart examines them in relation to the issues with their consumption.

Saccharine	(brand name: Sweet'N Low) Saccharine is 300 times as sweet as sugar. The oldest FDA-approved sweetener in widespread use, saccharine has undergone many trials and tests. The accusations of causing cancer haven't been proven, but all four negatives listed above are true for saccharine. Plus, it has a specific taste that most people can't stand.

Aspartame	(Equal or NutraSweet) Aspartame is 160 times as sweet as sugar. It is more expensive than saccharine, but it has a better taste. People with advanced liver disease or PKU (phenylketonuria) should never use aspartame. The sweet taste of aspartame is lost during cooking, so do not use it in place of sugar in recipes. Many scientific studies also point out a connection between aspartame and degenerative diseases like Alzheimer's and Parkinson's.
Sucralose	(Splenda) Sucralose is 600 times as sweet as sugar. As it is the newest AS, studies are currently being conducted to judge its safety. It is commonly used in cooking because it doesn't break down from heat.
Stevia	Stevia is 30 times sweeter than sugar. It is a naturally derived sweetener, produced from a plant native to Paraguay that has been used as a sweetener and flavor enhancer for centuries. A focal point of intrigue in recent years, Stevia is now sold legally in the United States but only as a "dietary supplement." You can find it in multiple forms at health food stores and grocers such as Trader Joe's and Whole Foods. It is heat stable, and there are many recipes using it that can be found online. No significant research has connected stevia to any diseases, but, like other sweeteners, overuse may still confuse the receptors in your brain.

Many sugar alcohols (such as xylitol, sorbitol, mannitol, maltitol) have been used for decades, frequently in gums or mints. While not calorie-free, they contain significantly fewer calories than sugar and are derived from the naturally occurring sugars of plants and fruits.

Sugar alcohols provide 1-3 calories per gram and are okay to use as long as those calories are acknowledged.

Although it lacks the low-calorie appeal of its counterparts, there is no reason to overlook sugar. Remember, sugar is a natural product and one that our body is able to metabolize from birth. One teaspoon of sugar is only 20 calories and requires very little insulin. However, when you are using sugar in a recipe, try cutting the amount down by one half to one third. You'll be surprised at how little you'll miss it.

* * *

22. Eating cheap doesn't pay off

Eating on a budget in no way means eating bad/cheap food. Unfortunately, many are eating fast and processed food because it's cheaper. Foods like fruits, vegetables, and lean protein that are recommended as a healthy choices cost more than a whole meal at a fast-food joint. The same is true for packaged and processed foods. Those last forever on the shelves and easily turn into human fat. Statistics show that low-income individuals are significantly more likely to be overweight. Government-offered "brown bags" usually contain muffins, bread, potatoes, and canned and packaged food. Cheap foods come in large quantities and poor quality and are dense in calories, mostly from fat and sugar, and low in healthy nutrients and vitamins. Habitual eating of fast, energy-dense foods eventually will cause weight gain and also make the person susceptible to other medical conditions and illnesses, such as sleep apnea, joint pains, low energy, and depression.

Unfortunately, our government subsidizes farming of crops like soy and corn that are used to create cheap foods. Hunger and obesity coincide in 37 million impoverished Americans. The World Health Organization is now characterizing obesity as one of the forms of malnutrition. With obesity, it's not the traditional meaning of not enough calories and nutrition, but too many calories and not enough nutrition

The immediate effect of eating fast food is also quite detrimental. Nothing is wrong with the actual process of eating—it's actually a lot of fun, particularly if you are a fast-food lover/addict. But even those people get the aftershock of a large, greasy, sugary meal—heartburn, sleepiness, and the blues. Want proof? Watch the film *Super Size Me*, by Morgan Spurlock.

Fast and cheap food is not just bad for your immediate and long-term health; it is also detrimental to our environment.

In his book *The Value of Nothing*, Raj Patel eloquently demonstrated that the social cost of a fast-food hamburger is $200. Surprised? When you look into all the future medical, ecological, and political disasters that the quarter pound of meat (meatlike substance) can result in, you will find the true cost of fast food. Every year in the United States of America, $100 billion is spent on obesity and related diseases. Internationally, fast food destroys local farming. The cost for the environment is very high. Eat locally grown food and support your local farmers. You'll save money on your health and save the environment.

* * *

23. Unconscious eating vs. food addiction

No person became overweight because he or she wanted it. No person ever desires to eat copious amounts of food, but many do it without planning or wanting. Weight gain happens on its own without the person's wish or control. While the overeater may be totally oblivious of his or her behavior, eventually the result becomes obvious. Weight goes up at some point and the pants don't fit, the seats seem to be smaller, the skirt is too tight, and only XXL T-shirts fit comfortably. How does it happen that when we need our mind, it seems deaf and mute to any self-control signals?

Most overweight people are not food addicts. They overeat because they do not pay attention, do not have enough knowledge, and do not try enough to keep their weight under control. But some people might have a food addiction. When food is eaten with the understanding that it is harmful in excess, it is called food abuse. Excess eating and craving for food constitutes a food addiction. It's hard to compare food with alcohol, cigarettes, or other drugs because we can live happily without those, but we can't live without food. On the other hand, more and more there is talk about food addiction and similarities with other addictions. There is plenty of scientific evidence that the same centers in the brain and the same neurotransmitters are involved.

Advances in brain imaging have enabled researchers to see inside the brains of addicts and patients with addictive behaviors. They can see in real time what gets people hooked: how the brain's reward system—based largely on the neurotransmitter dopamine—yearns for more, while inhibitory control centers, located in the frontal lobes, experience a system failure. Dr. Levounis, director of the Addiction Institute of New York at St. Luke's and Roosevelt Hospitals in Manhattan, talks about the ability of addictive substances, including food, to "hijack" the reward system of the brain.

Here is the normal formula: pleasure plus memory equals looking for more pleasure. Frontal lobes in a normally functioning brain are responsible for executive functioning and control, and they oversee the pleasure so that it does not turn into addiction. This is also known as willpower. Many things people like to do, like eating, exercising, and sex, follow this formula. In addicts, the addictive substance, like alcohol, heroin, cocaine, or food, takes over ("hijacks") the reward system, and the inhibition is not powerful enough to stop the craving.

Some morbidly obese people are certainly food addicts. That is likely also genetically predisposed. But many foods can provoke and create food or certain substance addiction. Common culprits are sugar, sweet tastes, diet drinks, coffee, caffeine, fast food, chocolate, and white bread, and some are unique. Have you ever heard of someone being addicted to broccoli or kale, or even carrots and apples? Fibrous foods are antidotes to addiction, while sweetness and fatness are promoters.

24. Emotional eating

Emotional eating is the practice of consuming large quantities of food—usually "comfort" or junk foods—in response to certain feelings, instead of as a response to hunger. Experts estimate that 75% of overeating is caused by emotions. Everyone knows food brings comfort, at least in the short term. As a result, people often turn to food to heal emotional problems. Eating becomes a habit preventing us from learning skills that can effectively resolve our emotional distress.

Depression, boredom, loneliness, chronic anger, anxiety, frustration, stress, problems with interpersonal relationships, and poor self-esteem can result in overeating and unwanted weight gain. By identifying what triggers the emotional eating, we can substitute more appropriate techniques to manage our emotional problems and take food and weight gain out of the equation.

How to Identify Eating Triggers

Situations and emotions that trigger comfort eating fall into six main categories.

- **Social.** Eating when around other people. For example, excessive eating can result from being encouraged by others to eat; eating to fit in; arguing; or feelings of inadequacy around other people.
- **Emotional.** Eating in response to boredom, stress, fatigue, tension, depression, anger, anxiety, or loneliness as a way to "fill the void."
- **Situational.** Eating because the opportunity is there. For example, at a restaurant, seeing an advertisement for a particular food,

passing by a bakery. Eating may also be associated with certain activities such as watching TV, going to the movies or a sporting event, etc.

- **Thoughts.** Eating as a result of negative self-worth or making excuses for eating. For example, scolding oneself for one's looks or a lack of willpower.
- **Physiological.** Eating in response to physical cues. For example, increased hunger due to skipping meals or eating to cure headaches or other pain.
- **Cultural.** In many cultures (it's true for my culture), refusing to taste the food prepared for you is considered an insult. People force their guests into eating, and the guests try every meal offered to them.

To identify what triggers excessive eating for you, keep a food diary that records what and when you eat as well as what stressors, thoughts, or emotions you identify as you eat. You should begin to identify patterns to your excessive eating fairly quickly.

25. Food politics

The politics of food, like any other politics, is dirty. Food politics can be thought about, for starters, as the practice of using food to influence behavior. There are many reasons to control the demand, production, transportation, advertisement, sales, and consumption of food. Comedian Jon Stewart put forth this comment about increasing government regulation: "Funding for regulatory agencies? Please. Now if you'll excuse me, I have a peanut butter, spinach, tomato, and Chinese toy sandwich to finish."

Marion Nestle's work *Food Politics* is subtitled *How the Food Industry Influences Nutrition and Health*. While the topic is indeed bigger than influential decisions made by the food industry, Nestle's work teaches us quite a lot.

To stay away from ugly food politics, we need to stay close to our local farmers. Most all the food you can buy at a farmer's market is healthy. The exceptions are the cookies, but even those are okay when eaten in small quantities. Some culprits of obesity, like high fructose corn syrup, cannot even be found at farmer's markets, because only big food corporations are able to buy it. Most other culprits, like trans fats, salt, and artificial sweeteners, are also not popular among the farmers, because all they sell is real food. There is some packaged food, but it has quite a short half-life. The shopping experience at a farmer's market is also not to miss. Farmer's markets are more environmentally healthy. The carbon footprint of our food is measured in terms of petroleum used to plant, fertilize, harvest, and transport our crops. Crops produced locally are more likely to be sold while in season, but sometimes are more expensive as they do not exploit the cheap labor found overseas. Your local farmers have the best food of all. Check online for farmer's markets near you at www. localharvest.org.

* * *

26. The impact of the environment on weight

The environment's impact on weight starts in childhood and continues at any age and social status. Our society, on one hand, constantly talks about obesity, and, on the other hand, it creates an obesogenic (obesity-creating) environment. We are a big part of it. Starting from childhood, our environment has plenty of unhealthy offerings that mostly are picked by people with genes predisposed to be drawn to those foods. Our environment affects us not only genetically, but in most every way.

- "Eat, finish your plate, think of starving poor children," we are told as children.
- Numerous birthday parties at preschool and school, vending machines at school, cheap fast food, and extra-large-size sodas in high school, too much pizza and doughnuts in college.
- People work for hours glued to their computers, and the only exercise they get is to walk to the break room to have coffee, cookies, doughnuts, M&Ms, or, at best, a fruit-flavored yogurt full of high fructose corn syrup.
- Going to a movie and sitting for two hours while getting 1,200 calories from soda and buttered popcorn is a part of our culture.
- TV is one of the culprits. It's addictive and has multiple seductive food ads that confuse the mind. TV ads for cheap restaurants or sugary snacks show smiling faces that are as fabricated as a laugh track.

- Fast food is cheap, flavorful, and addictive—plus customers need not even get out of their cars to get a 1,000-calorie meal.
- Even the coffee shops turned into calorie-offering machines. They also serve pies laden with trans fats, but of course they are not labeled as such.
- Holidays like Fourth of July, Labor Day, Thanksgiving, and, of course, Christmas are considered to be a legitimate reason to gain several pounds.
- We fear being rude if we refuse the desserts brought to social functions while we know most contain partially hydrogenated oils, HFCS, or simply too much sugar.

Frequently people fully understand the impact of the environmental culprits but do not care to be the ones to make the change. Change is hard work. Inertia is easy. Who should be the one to stop bringing doughnuts to study rooms? Who should suggest that other students stop bringing doughnuts? Several studies have shown that when people are surrounded with stores that carry healthy foods, the prevalence of obesity goes down.

* * *

27. Americans at low cardiac risk are a vanishing breed

People in the age group from 25 to 74 with low risk for heart disease now make up less than 8% of the U.S. population.

Persons with a low-risk-factor burden met these criteria: not currently smoking; total cholesterol less than 200 mg/dL; not using lipid-lowering medications; systolic blood pressure less than 120 mm Hg and diastolic blood pressure less than 80 mm Hg; not using antihypertensive medications; body mass index less than 25 kg/m^2; and not having been previously diagnosed with diabetes. So, the rest of the population or 92% of people ages 25 to 74, in the United States of America, is out of shape, hypertensive, has high cholesterol, smokes, or has diabetes. Doesn't this make you heartsick? This pattern was the same for men and women. Whites were more likely to be living heart-healthy lives than were blacks, but that didn't make the total number higher than 8%. Europeans do better with their weight but have more smokers, so the percentages of "healthy" people in Europe are not much different.

Now, some out of the 92% with a high risk will have a pure genetic predisposition for excess weight, diabetes, hypertension, or high cholesterol, but many or most will develop these risk factors with the help of poor lifestyle habits. Many studies have shown that diabetes is preventable when people work on their eating habits, increase activity, and lose weight. Most of you are younger than 25 and this survey doesn't apply to you—at least not yet. But by improving your lifestyle, you can prevent these epidemiological disasters and stay in the low-cardiac-risk group. You are responsible for improving this tragic ratio. Prevention is easier, cheaper, and more rewarding.

* * *

28. Is thin the new happy?

The answer is absolutely no. Valerie Frankel, in her book *Thin is the New Happy*, gives compelling evidence against the title of her own book. "No food tastes better than skinny," said Kate Moss, and her image as a model is far from happiness. Many celebrities are skinny; most have to work very, very hard to be like that. Many models and actresses at some point came out of the closet and confessed to being anorectic or bulimic. Being skinny or thin can't bring you happiness or health, but being normal weight or liking your body at whatever weight you're at can take your mind off your own body image. Starving and vomiting to look thinner or prettier makes no sense but happens all the time.

Almost every woman after 40 would agree that she would like to be thinner. No wonder 85 million people in this country are dieting. In the healthy category of women, the only ones who do not need to lose weight are the ones who work out religiously and control their eating habits. Among 20-year-olds there are many girls who do not need to lose weight; so far, without much effort, they are naturally thin. A good start, though, doesn't mean a lifetime achievement of a perfect weight. The metabolism goes down, mobility decreases, and if the normal-weight girl doesn't exercise or eat healthy, the weight gain happens despite the good start and the good genes. The same is true for boys. If, during college, the biggest contributor to weight gain for boys is the alcohol, later in life it's the sedentary lifestyle and oblivion to the quantity or the quality of food that is being consumed.

Being thin is not going to make you happy, but having control over your weight will save you a lot of doctor's visits, pill taking, and undergoing multiple procedures to test for complications of obesity.

* * *

29. "You have diabetes"

These are the words anyone dreads to hear. Some young people have already heard those words, but their diabetes, known as type 1, has no connection to food. Type 1 diabetes occurs in young people who have the predisposing genetic makeup and get hit by the virus that can turn on those genes. But the vast majority of people suffering from diabetes have type 2 diabetes, which is attributed to their poor lifestyle. Ninety percent of those can prevent this lifelong disease if only they watch what they eat and exercise regularly. More and more, type 2 diabetes is diagnosed in younger adults, something that was almost unheard of 30 years ago. Half of all diabetics under age 20 have type 2 diabetes.

In 2011, epidemiologic studies estimated there are about 25.8 million diabetics in the United States. Ten years ago, the same studies estimated there were only 16 million diabetics. Today there are about 300 million people in the world with diabetes. In the United States we have about 4.5% of the world's population and about 8.5 % of all of the diabetics. There is only one answer to this discrepancy—the American lifestyle.

Thirty years of the intensive Western lifestyle and the population is suffering from the obesity pandemic that in many evolves into diabetes. We have witnessed another new phenomenon thanks to our obesity epidemic: in some people diabetes goes away, just like a cold or pneumonia. Here is how: people who get gastric bypass surgery and lose a lot of weight often see their diabetes vanish. So for some, diabetes is actually a curable disease. Any doctor 30 years ago would call it a bluff, but today it's possible. There is another, much healthier process to get the same result—it's called "Don't get obese in the first place."

* * *

Part 2.
The Alpha Plan

A few minutes spent searching the Internet or perusing celebrity magazines will reveal innumerable fad diets on the market. Be they Dukan, Atkins, South Beach, Flat Belly, Mediterranean, Cabbage Soup, Astronaut's, or Coconut diets, all of these and more will be tried time and time again by millions of consumers. So how is the Alpha Diet unique?

All of the above diets focus on losing weight by eliminating or emphasizing certain foods. The Alpha Diet is the first diet that teaches you how not to gain the weight in the first place. The Alpha Plan is a healthy lifestyle that combines the Alpha Diet and conscious physically active behavior. College is the right time to start. Your 20s and 30s are a great time to make the change. The Alpha Diet could be seen as a constitution for governing your health. Complying with the amendments of the Alpha Diet is a great way of investing into your health and avoiding a slew of metabolic diseases.

Welcome the change

> *"We must always change, renew, rejuvenate ourselves, otherwise we harden."*
>
> **Goethe**

Humans are creatures of habit. Some habits we have to lose and some we have to gain and accept. Healthy eating and regular exercising eventually grows on you, but you need to give it a chance. Here is an obvious example: start eating breakfast. If you force yourself to eat breakfast for two weeks in a row, it will grow on you and most likely will turn into a habit. Try the variety of breakfasts in this book—they are all extremely tasty and, of course, healthy. "I hate vegetables," "I hate eggplant," "I hate all the fruits except for bananas"—these kinds of comments come out of the mouths of people of all ages, but mostly children and teens. You might not like everything new that you try, but some new things will appeal to you and you will incorporate them into your daily living. Avoid being dogmatic not only in regard to food but also everything else in life.

If you can't cook, you should learn

"When we no longer have good cooking in the world, we will have no literature, nor high and sharp intelligence, nor friendly gathering, nor social harmony."

Marie-Antoine Careme

Mageirocophobia is a fear of cooking. Some people have a fear of cooking for large groups; others just have a fear of touching a raw egg or meat. But most people are either lazy or were never taught to cook. Not cooking has been simplified and rewarded by our society. We are surrounded with a variety of packaged meals, frozen dinners, and inexpensive restaurants. Eating those meals is quick, unadventurous, and far away from using creativity and imagination.

Cooking is a great pleasure and is a way to completely avoid the bad ingredients used by the food industry. When you cook regularly, you also learn to appreciate good food and the work of professional chefs. Then you can truly enjoy a beautiful meal in front of you in a restaurant. Fast-food chains don't have chefs, they have managers. What you eat is not art but a corporate product, an imitation of food.

The Common Sense and Capability of Practicing Moderation

"Moderation is an ostentatious proof of our strength of character. To eat is a necessity, but to eat intelligently is an art."

Francois de La Rochefoucauld

Not many achieve this virtuous ability, but all should strive when it comes to things like food, alcohol, and quite a few other matters. If moderation is the mechanism for achieving a successful, healthy lifestyle, then common sense is the theory behind it. Common sense, otherwise known as sound judgment, is frequently missing in people of all ages. It's a knowledge that usually grows with experience, but sometimes it doesn't. As a result, some can finish a whole pie, two burgers with fries, a twelve-pack of beer, or a bottle of vodka, or smoke marijuana daily. When common sense and the ability to practice moderation are damaged, the person gets addicted to the certain vice and becomes an alcoholic, food addict, sugar addict, pot-head, etc. In those conditions, professional help may be necessary.

Look around, look into the mirror, and try to look into your future. You certainly have to figure out how to eat and drink in moderation and enjoy life as it is.

Be friendly to the environment: eat seasonal, locally grown food

"There is a sufficiency in the world for man's need but not for man's greed."

Gandhi

The way we eat impacts the environment and our domestic and world economy. The industrialization of food comes at a high cost to our ecology. Food marketing, most of which promotes weight gain, spends $32 billion per year. Most packaging is made from oil, and a vast majority of those colorful plastics end up in landfills for hundreds of years. Thanks to the glamour of the Western supermarket, we are no longer confined to the fruit and vegetable seasonal limits. Whether it's the middle of the winter or in the middle of the summer we can buy exactly the same produce. But why do we need to be so complacent or greedy that we need strawberries, bananas, tomatoes, and grapes year round? In the wrong season, produce is grown thousands of miles away, picked very green, sprayed with strong wrinkle-preventing chemicals, and then flown to us on jumbo carbon-emitting airplanes so we do not forget what they look like for the eight months they aren't grown locally. Instead, you should eat the variety of foods available at your local market. This eliminates the need for the child labor, chemicals, and airplanes used for transporting food to places where there is plenty of food already.

Eating becomes a political act.

Love what you see in the mirror

"You, yourself, as much as anybody in the entire universe, deserve your love and affection."

Buddha

Poor body image, as some girls and women have, is a cause of weight gain. Ignoring the body image, as some boys and men do, also results in weight gain. There is only one body and one face that you've inherited from your genes and environment. Take it or leave it. Or, there is a better option – take it and do your best with it. Loving yourself means taking good care of you.

"It is not the mountain we conquer but ourselves."

Edmund Hillary

Know how to laugh at yourself

"Humor is mankind's greatest blessing."

Mark Twain

Humor saves lives. Logical thinking prevents many mistakes and often leads to success. Unfortunately, logic doesn't always work. Humor helps one cope in those situations where reason fails. Humor is one of the tools to achieve self-confidence. Self-effacing humor is usually a sign of confidence. Being able to laugh at yourself is a good sign of a positive mind-set.

If you have excess weight, too much stress, bad luck, and unfriendly genes, then to survive and to make the best of it you need a sense of humor. Humor is a practical way to turn any painful situation around. It works as an antidote to pain, stress, and conflict. Using humor and laughter can balance out the frustrations of weight loss. Laughter has a healing force and, of course, is the best medicine.

1. Read labels

Reading labels takes time and patience, but in general it's not rocket science. Every package of food contains quite a bit of information. Unfortunately, many of the labels are encrypted by the manufacturers. Certain phrases such as "All Natural," "Healthy," "Excellent source of fiber," "0g Trans Fats," "Low Fat," and "Low Carb" are all there to lure and confuse the customer. With a little training, you will be able to spot the facts and fallacies.

To begin, every label has two important concepts that you need to know: nutrition facts and ingredients.

Nutrition facts: This is where you learn about the types and amounts of fats, cholesterol, protein, carbohydrates, sugar, and fiber per serving. Serving size and calorie count are a part of nutrition facts.

a) **Serving size**—Frequently, people read the carbohydrate or fat content of a food product and are misled. The serving size is the quantity of food consumed in one serving, or what the manufacturers deem as one serving. The calorie count and nutrient amount are presented as one serving, not for the whole of the product.

b) **Calorie count**—The total number of calories per serving. Watch out for the serving size. For example, five crackers is the serving size that has the 100 calories, not the whole bag; the whole bag may have seven servings.

When reading Nutrition Facts, pay attention to the following:

Nutrition Facts

Serving Size 1 cup (228g)
Servings Per Container 2

Amount Per Serving

Calories 250   Calories from Fat 110

	% Daily Value*
Total Fat 12g	**18%**
Saturated Fat 3g	**15%**
Trans Fat 3g	
Cholesterol 30mg	**10%**
Sodium 470mg	**20%**
Total Carbohydrate 31g	**10%**
Dietary Fiber 0g	**0%**
Sugars 5g	
Protein 5g	

Vitamin A	4%
Vitamin C	2%
Calcium	20%
Iron	4%

* Percent Daily Values are based on a 2,000 calorie diet. Your Daily Values may be higher or lower depending on your calorie needs.

	Calories	2,000	2,500
Total Fat	Less than	65g	80g
Sat Fat	Less than	20g	25g
Cholesterol	Less than	300mg	300mg
Sodium	Less than	2,400mg	2,400mg
Total Carbohydrate		300g	375g
Dietary Fiber		25g	30g

- **Always find the serving size at the top of the label.**
- **Decide on how much you will eat.**
- **Find the total carbohydrates per serving.** In this particular case, bagels have a large amount of carbohydrates, so a half bagel might be all you should eat.
- **Dietary fiber and sugar form the sum of total carbohydrates.** When buying cereal, get one that has more than 4 grams of fiber and no more than 10 grams of sugar in one serving of cereal. The more fiber and the less sugar, the healthier is your cereal. The total carbohydrate count is less important. Foods rich in fiber slow the digestion of carbohydrates, require less insulin and keep the person fuller for longer periods of time.
- **Pay attention to the fat amount/type and the protein amount.** It's not important if you are eating a bagel but very important if you

are choosing a type of meat or cookies. When buying cereals, try to find one with around 4 grams or more of protein per serving.

* * *

2. Recognize the ingredients

Reading the ingredients on the labels can help you to understand what it is that you are putting in your mouth. Remember the simple formula: your health depends on the type of food and the amount of food you eat. If the food is loaded with artificial chemicals such as trans fats, high fructose corn syrup, and other nasty additives, just put it back on the shelf. If the ingredient list is long and complicated, as it is for coffee creamer or many white breads, that is usually a sign that your meal is chock-full of heavy chemicals; that is the type you need to avoid. As a rule, if the ingredient list is longer than five lines, the product is not going to be good for you. You will notice that sugar and cholesterol are not listed as ingredients to be avoided. While both can induce disease when consumed in large amounts, both are natural products and in small amounts are harmless. The ingredients to avoid are man made and may contribute to illness even in small amounts. Here are the four ubiquitous ingredients to be avoided:

1. Partially hydrogenated oil, an artificial substance also known as vegetable shortening, margarine, or trans fat. After decades of usage, trans-fats have only recently been acknowledged for their evil properties but still are plentiful on the market.
2. High fructose corn syrup (HFCS) is a highly processed substance, used in place of sweeteners.
3. Artificial sweeteners like saccharine, aspartame, or sucralose (AS) are used in products labeled "no sugar" or "no calorie."

4. Food coloring like Yellow #5, Yellow #6, Blue #2 or #1, Red #3 or #40, or others, and artificial flavorings.

None of those ingredients belongs in your food. All of these are artificially made substances produced to sell and preserve foods; they all promote weight gain, and they are all enemies of a healthy life-style.

* * *

3. Snacking: a friend or a foe?

One of the answers to French slimness is no snacking. No snacking explains the "French paradox": the French eat foie gras, chocolate, cheese, bread, drink lots of wine, yet they stay slim. So, if one can eat three meals a day and stay away from snacks, great! However, don't starve yourself and then jump at food and overeat. If the meals are truly nutritious and contain proportional amounts of carbohydrates, protein, and fat, then the eater will stay full for five to six hours until his or her next meal. A good example of a French breakfast is a butter croissant and a cup of coffee with cream; simple, yet satisfying, with a total of 380 calories, 23 grams of fat, 6 grams of protein, and 37 grams of carbohydrate.

Americans love snacks. From a young age, we are programmed to have snacks. Children, students, and adults grab a cookie after lunch not because they're still hungry, but because they're used to it. As a result, the appetite-affecting hormones like leptin, GLP-1, and ghrelin are either over activated because the snack is too sugary or they are resistant because the person is already overweight.

Not all snacking, however, is bad for you—just the snacks that come from vending machines, the middle sections of supermarkets, and movie theatres. There is some smart snacking, sometimes even necessary snacking. There are several scenarios when snacks are good for you—for example, if you haven't eaten for three or four hours and are heading to the gym. Before exercising, snacking can help you build muscle, versus losing it. A great pre-workout snack is a banana and milk, a healthy food bar, or a peanut butter sandwich and a big glass of water.

Here are some examples of healthy snacks; raw vegetables (to be eaten any time and in large portions), whole-grain crackers (about six) and low-fat cheese, a handful of nuts, dark chocolate, plain yogurt with berries or other fruit, popcorn with a pinch of salt, and an oatmeal or chocolate chip cookie that is under 200 calories.

* * *

4. Drink plenty of water

We are made of water. Seventy percent of our body, 80% of our blood, and 85% of our gray matter is made of water, and we need it to survive, function, and stay healthy. This is a known fact, so it is kind of surprising to learn that most people are not drinking enough water. Thirst can be interpreted as hunger by the tired brain. There is also correlation between weight and insufficient water drinking. So, do yourself a favor. Drink lots of water. Remember, we constantly lose water—obviously through "number one", but also through breathing and our skin. It's estimated that we lose about 10 cups of water on a hot day without any major activity. We need to replenish it through water and other liquids like soups, fruits, vegetables, tea, coffee, and mineral water. Soda is not water. It makes you thirsty and hungry. Both types of sodas, regular and diet, promote obesity and diabetes, and there is ample evidence to support their harmful effects. What about juices? Too much sugar (*even in no-sugar-added juice*) and no fiber. So forget the juice; eat the fruit and drink the water. Having said all that, if you're not fighting your weight, then real fruit juice is fine, but make sure it's not daily or many times per day. The best thing about water is that it lacks calories, fills you up, and hydrates you to make your body functions smooth. Here are some commonly asked questions, answered.

Q. What kind of water should you drink?
A. Any kind: bottled, filtered, from the faucet, from the water-cooler, at school, at work, or in a store.
Q. How much water should you drink?

A. On a hot day, a minimum of five cups of water per day. The rest should be mineral water, tea, coffee, soup, and occasionally juice. If the weather is moderate then 6-8 cups of total fluid would suffice.

Q. What is the best kind of fluid to drink?

A. Water is always good; you can't go wrong with it. But if you are bored, then the other choices include these:

- Black coffee is great with or after breakfast. Avoid drinking more than three cups per day. Use as little cream as possible. Coffee has multiple beneficial effects.
- Black tea is great. Green tea is even better and has some appetite-suppressant effects, just like coffee has antioxidant ability.
- Mineral, natural-flavored, and carbonated water is great for those who like bubbles. A very good habit is to drink water half an hour before meals—fills up the stomach.

Q. Should you drink water all day long?

A. No! Don't drink water two hours before getting into bed unless you're thirsty. Drink your water before meals and between meals.

* * *

5. Sleep to be healthy

College and sleep don't get along together for some students. First, there is no one to chase them or even suggest to them to go to bed, and second, there are too many distractions, like friends, computers, homework, eating, drinking, studying, partying, and more. In one large study, more than 50% of fall-asleep crashes involved drivers 25 or younger.

It's proven that sleep makes a great difference in weight management. Turns out that Americans have been sleeping about two hours less than 40 years ago, and that also contributes to the epidemic of obesity. A survey by the American Cancer Society found that the average American was sleeping eight or nine hours per night in 1960, and that dropped to seven hours by 1995. Today, about 30% of adults sleep fewer than six hours a night. Sleep deprivation influences our weight through several mechanisms. The most obvious mechanism is that the longer you are awake, the hungrier you get and the more you eat. Other reasons are more scientific:

- During sleep we have a change in most hormones, including the ones that influence satiety (fullness) and the appetite. During sleep, the satiety hormone leptin goes down, and when people are sleep deprived, leptin resistance occurs and hunger increases.
- Sleep-restricted people crave mostly carbohydrates, sugars, and calorie-dense foods.
- Sleep deprivation leads to insulin resistance, and that helps you build up the fat around your stomach and eventually, in predisposed people, diabetes develops.

A minimum of eight hours of sleep is shown to maintain a healthy weight, keep you happy, and prolong longevity. Develop a healthy habit: turn off the computer and the TV no later than 11 p.m. Reading a nonfiction or homework-related book in bed will help you to fall asleep more easily than you think. Avoid reading a horror or a mystery novel or anything that Is hard to put down.

* * *

6. Avoid all sodas and most fruit juices

If you don't have excess weight and don't want any then try to use sweet-tasting drinks sparingly. If you are gaining weight and need to lose it, then it's a good idea to avoid all regular and diet sodas, as well as fruit juices.

Portion control will turn into an impossible effort if you ignore this suggestion. Why? The large amount of sugar in regular sodas and fruit juices stimulates insulin secretion by the pancreas. The over secreted insulin puts sugar into the muscles or liver and drops blood sugar lower. This creates the more need for sugar, initiating a vicious circle. The high fructose corn syrup (HFCS) in soda and fructose in fruit juices act on the brain, lowering the satiety sensation. These pathways explain why the more you drink, the more you want to drink and eat.

Diet sodas act by a different mechanism. A diet soda drinker gets used to the *sweet* (even artificially sweet) taste of the soda and looks for more of that same sweetness. It has been shown that diet soda drinkers consume more calories than regular soda drinkers, almost like their brain gives them a green light for more food because the fake sweetness in the drink did not deliver the promised calories.

Water, tea, and mineral waters are what you need to stay hydrated. One or two cups of coffee a day are also okay. Sugary drinks are okay only when you exercise hard and regularly.

Results from a large study done on 71,000 American nurses showed that consumption of vegetables and fruits was associated with less diabetes and obesity, and drinking juice turned out to be a risk factor for both of those.

* * *

7. Eat breakfast daily

A lot of people skip breakfast. Let's call them "skippers." A skipper doesn't have time and he has not been used to eating breakfast since childhood. Rarely does he grab a cup of fancy coffee at Starbucks on his way to school; on most days he eats nothing.

Many of the "skippers" end up overweight. Not eating breakfast usually sets the person up to impulsively snack throughout the day, often on high-fat sweets and then eating extra servings or bigger portions at lunch or dinner. Time is very important at any age. A couple more minutes of sleep is very precious when you went to bed at 3 a.m. Nevertheless, it pays to make time for what may be the most important meal of the day. According to some studies, eating the right breakfast every day may reduce the risk for obesity and insulin resistance—an early sign of developing diabetes—by as much as 35% to 50%.

Try to choose foods from at least two or more food groups. Protein foods take longer to digest and will provide sustained energy and keep you feeling full longer. Here are quick, tasty, and nutritious choices to get your day off to a good start: whole-grain cereals (look for ones with more than 5 grams of protein and more than 5 grams of fiber per serving) with 2% or whole milk and 10 almonds; a smoothie with protein and fruit; energy bars like Luna or Clif bars or others. Read the labels. Make sure the bar is free of high fructose corn syrup (HFCS), partially hydrogenated fats, food coloring, or artificial sweeteners (AS). Coffee, tea, milk, and soy milk are all great and should be a part of your breakfast. When eating breakfast, protein is essential to keep your appetite under control. In Part 4 there are a variety of easy-to-make breakfasts for college or any time after.

* * *

8. Eat organic when you can

Why eat organic? Organic food, by its legal definition, is food from plants and animals that is produced without chemical or synthetic additives or pesticides. And, according to the National Center for Appropriate Technology, organic farming helps retain water in the soil, producing more drought-resistant crops.

A study from Washington University demonstrated that children eating mostly organic food had lower levels of organophosphorus (OP) than those who ate conventionally grown foods. Studies suggest that chronic low-level exposure to OP pesticides may affect neurological functioning, neurodevelopment, and growth in children.

However, there is a disadvantage to an organic lifestyle: the price of the food. Organic produce is about 50% more costly than its conventional counterpart, and meat and milk are even more expensive. Organic farming requires more skill and produces a smaller bounty than conventional methods, leading to a sharp price increase.

Realistically, it's difficult to buy only organic food, especially on the tight college budget. And, with certain foods, it's fine to save some money and buy the conventional variety. Before you buy, consider a few factors, including how many permeable surfaces the food has (for example, something leafy like lettuce is very permeable to chemicals) and how much spraying and irrigation it requires. It is particularly important to choose the organic forms of foods like strawberries, watermelons, artichokes, potatoes, peanut butter, milk, meat, tofu, and coffee.

Remember, just because you can find the word "organic" somewhere on your food wrapper doesn't mean it's 100% organic. The USDA regulates terms on organic food labels:

- "100% Organic"—The food comes from a regularly inspected organic grower/importer and has no synthetic ingredients. Has a seal of authenticity.
- "Organic"—Food that has a minimum of 95% organic ingredients can qualify for this seal.
- "Made with Organic Ingredients"—The food must contain at least 70% organic ingredients and can list them on the front.
- For foods that have less than 70% organic ingredients, they may list any organic ingredients on the side.
- Meat, eggs, poultry, and dairy labeled "organic" must come from animals that have never received antibiotics or growth hormones. There are no set standards for organic seafood.

With the recent popularity of the "green food" movement, the organic food industry has propagated into a monstrously big business. Most organic brands today are linked to the same companies that rejected organic processes before, but eventually turned to the organic label to attract customers. Over time, the definition of "organic" has changed as well. Years ago, it simply meant locally grown food without pesticides or chemicals, while today it means a label with a USDA stamp. In some circumstances, a cow that produces organic milk might never see the light of day.

How can you distinguish *good organic* from *bad organic*? Clearly, there are other parameters by which food can be measured. Organic production stickers assure the absence of pesticides, unnatural fertilizers, and genetically modified organisms, but one must also look for products supplied by "free-range or pastured" animals, and also consider the reduced carbon footprint of locally transported foods, as well as the task of choosing foods made without excess sugars or ugly additives. Yes, the cost is slightly higher than your name-brand childhood favorites. But, for the sake of the environment and your own health, a few extra dollars is a small price to pay.

* * *

9. Balancing willpower

"Most powerful is he who has himself in his own power."

Seneca

Wikipedia explains "willpower" as self-control, or the ability of a person to exert his or her will over the inhibitions of his or her body or self. Willpower and weight loss have an intimate relationship. Weight loss is pretty much impossible without the heavy use of willpower.

To quote Madonna, "Sometimes you have to be a bitch to get things done." In the case of willpower, sometimes you have to be a bitch toward yourself. To achieve personal discipline, you need to be able to overcome those strong inner urges.

"I know that double-chocolate-chip cookie is bad for me, but I still want it." "I know exercise is good for me, but I can't force myself to get off the couch." Such is the inner fight between the easy yet destructive comfort otherwise known as instant gratification vs. the conscious behavior. This fight is filled with effort and action but is never satisfying immediately. The satisfaction arrives later, in the form of a healthy body and mind.

Truly, most people know why and how they gained the weight and they also know why they can't lose it. So, it's not just the understanding of the consequences and effects of the weight. It's about being able to use willpower to eat less and exercise more. Both major components of weight gain, excessive eating, and not exercising are consequences of weak willpower or lack of willpower.

Here is what happened with smoking in America, which is similar to excessive eating. Once people realized the harm caused by smoking, many quit—some more easily than others, but all of them had to use willpower. As a result of the major antismoking campaign, forty-years later, we still have 26.5% of the population smoking. Some of these people have no interest in quitting, but many want to quit and have a very hard time doing it, because they just do not have enough willpower. They say it's a nicotine addiction. Is it? What about the other 60%? How did they quit? After all, they also had nicotine receptors and the nicotine dependence. So, maybe the 60% had stronger and more effective willpower.

Now, here is the bad news: our willpower or self-control is fighting against the appetite regulation that is genetically programmed. Also, our willpower has to fight against all the technological conveniences and progress, like cars, remotes, escalators, elevators, computers, video games, TVs, movie theaters, etc. It was a lot easier for our great-grandparents, who had to walk to school in the next village every day and never heard of trans fats. Our willpower is forced into the unfair fight against all of the food industry ads and ubiquitous abundance of food.

Our willpower is powered by knowledge and government bans (unfortunately, those are sometimes necessary.) The lack of willpower, or "ill power," is fed by genes, the environment, hormones, neurotransmitters, and technology. I think that ill power and willpower are like Goofus and Gallant, or maybe even like the Joker and Batman. Never underestimate the Joker.

Here are several suggestions:
- Be nice to your willpower and don't abuse it.
- Just like with children, pick your battles. For a while, make exercise your priority, and try to get your 10,000 steps in every day of the week. Next week, take walks, but make your priority avoiding all the snacks, ice cream, desserts, cookies, candies, etc. The week after, do not eat anything after 6 p.m.
- Drink lots of water and get seven to eight hours of sleep each night, because willpower works better when you are hydrated and rested.

* * *

10. How to lose weight

The Alpha Plan is about healthy weight and the prevention of obesity. But it can be used as a tool to lose weight. Theoretically, losing weight is simple. All you need to do to lose weight is achieve a negative calorie balance. In other words, the calories that you consume through food should be less than the calories spent for the needs of the body, such as breathing, chewing, digesting, sleeping, the work of our hearts, otherwise known as basic metabolic rate (BMR), and physical activity. Simply put, you have to use more calories than you take in.

Weight loss = Δ in spent energy (BMR + energy used for daily activities and exercise) – consumed calories (food)

To solve this equation, you need to know the amount of both calories burned and calories consumed. First, you should calculate the number of calories you need daily for your body's basic function, known as your BMR, or basic metabolic rate. One easy way to find your BMR is to remember that for every pound that you weigh, your body burns 10 calories. So, if you are 150 pounds, your body burns 1,500 calories per day. BMR also adjusts with factors, including age, gender, and even height, that, for the sake of convenience, we will overlook.

In addition to facilitating metabolic functions, we need calories to support our physical activity. If you're sedentary, find 20% of your BMR and add it to your total. If your behavior is not sedentary but you don't exercise regularly, add 30%; if you're active, 40%. Also, about

100 calories are spent on digestion. So far, an average woman who exercises occasionally and weighs 130 pounds requires about 1,300 + 520 + 100 = 1,920 calories per day. For men, we need to add another 300 calories.

So, what happens with the rest of the consumed calories? The excess of calories leads to an accumulation of body fat, meaning it will either be stored or will prevent the mobilization and burning of endogenous (stored) fat. In general, ingesting 3,500 calories per week less than expended will lead to a loss of approximately 1 pound of fat. That is equal to 500 calories less per day.

Using your weight to find the calorie count for the day works when you have a normal or desired weight. For those with excess weight, the math should be done based on your ideal or desired weight.

Genetic factors may influence the amount of weight gained with overeating as well as the amount of weight lost with a negative calorie balance. Therefore, don't be surprised if your friend eats and exercises the same amount as you, yet loses more weight. It's likely due to changes in nonvolitional energy expenditure, which means things we can't control, such as fidgeting, that may be also determined genetically. The Alpha Plan does not require calorie counting, but you need to understand calories and certainly do the simple math if you need to lose weight. In reality there are many other factors, including genetics, age, sex hormones, and gut hormones. You have control only in regard to the energy and its balance.

To achieve weight loss or to avoid gaining weight, you need to learn the types and amount of food to eat and these foods' impact on your health. Avoiding calorie-dense foods in favor of nutritious foods is more important than tallying numbers. With time, healthy eating will become second nature and you will learn to dislike unhealthy foods. It is unheard of for healthy eaters to make a drastic change and become fast-food junkies. But it is also hard for people who love sweets and fried foods to transform into healthy eaters. Frequently, this transition is made on doctor's orders. Why wait for that?

* * *

11. Do you need to weigh?

Is it a good idea to step on a scale every now and then? It is! If you have a tendency to gain weight or already have excess weight, you want to own bathroom scales. Scales keep you grounded and enlighten you on how you are doing with your weight. Weigh yourself once a week or even every morning after taking a shower. About 2 to 3 pounds up and down is normal, but if you notice a consistent rise, it is a message to act. Go after the most obvious culprits—omit the nighttime ice cream, third slice of pizza, and sugary drinks. Small changes can prevent small rises in weight. Also, don't forget that the scale also encourages you to get off your duff and do something about those pounds.

If you're someone who is thin and exercising daily and all you worry about is getting the necessary calories to cover your heavy exercise, it's still a good idea to check on your weight to make sure you maintain it.

If you're someone who hates the scales and gets anxious every time you think about the scale, then forget it. Use the way your pants or skirt fit as a criteria. You know that you've lost weight when you need to go shopping for a smaller size. If your pants are tight and the buttons need adjustments, then instead of going shopping for a larger size or baggier clothes, it's time to revise your lifestyle. Pants, skirt, or bra tightness would work. Scales are a part of the Alpha Plan. It's useful and a good idea to own one even when you live in a dorm.

* * *

12. Enjoy your movie without packing on the pounds

Movies are notorious for the amount of calories consumed by oblivious moviegoers. People come to a movie theater to enjoy a movie, get distracted from their own issues, and enjoy the adventurous lives of the characters in the movie. The goal is certainly not to consume hundreds to thousands of calories but to enjoy the movie. Frequently it's also a social event. But even going to restaurants, sometimes people get fewer calories than at a movie.

It is a part of American tradition to get a large bucket of buttery popcorn (that has gotten tremendously large over the last 20 years), a sugary drink, and candy right before getting comfortable for about two hours of complete immobility. Then the viewer forgets about his or her own problems, including weight, and dives into the realm of Hollywood problems. The only connection with the world remains the bucket of popcorn, the candy, and the sugary drink to wash the fat and the salt down. The faster the pace of the movie, the faster people chew and get to another fistful of greasy popcorn or Milk Duds. People who buy all three best-seller junk foods at the theater—popcorn, candy, and soda—usually consume about 1,200–2,500 calories, 60 grams of saturated fat, 2,000 milligrams of sodium, and 20–35 teaspoons of sugar.

But why put the body through such trauma? "Because when you go to a movie you always get popcorn and an Icee!" was my son's answer when he was 10.

But the main calorie consumers are not 10. Many are adults with already present potbellies. If you're trying to eat healthy yet you go to the movies and consume a large portion of calories, even if it is only occasionally, that still could be the cause of the weight not coming down or even gaining weight.

Here is the solution. You can't afford the American movie snack tradition, so just get a small bottle of water (the large one will force you to spend some of the precious movie time in the bathroom) or chew gum. Why not unbuttered popcorn? Because at the theaters, all the popcorn comes from packages which have some oil, frequently partially hydrogenated oil, added to it. "Buttered" only means an additional butter is added to it. So, here is a novel thought: just enjoy the movie without adding another task like eating or drinking.

* * *

13. How to satisfy your sweet tooth

"Sweet tooth" is a commonly known term for a craving or difficulty resisting sweets. "Sugarholism" is probably another term for that, except for people who become aware about their craving for sweets at a lot younger age. Just like with alcohol, some people have an easier time controlling the sugar craving than others.

Sugar cravings are also typical for people with metabolic syndrome or insulin resistance syndrome. These are people with exaggerated production of insulin in response to sugar consumption. As a result of overproduction of insulin, blood sugar drops and the person experiences hypoglycemia, which requires more sugar ingestion. It's not surprising that these people are more prone to developing diabetes. Most people who have a sweet tooth and can't control it after ages 40 (if not younger) eventually gain some excess weight.

As a society, ours does a lot to promote the sweet tooth and provoke the sugar cravings: birthday cakes and juice for every child in preschool, vending machines, Halloween candy, large soft drinks, malt balls, M&Ms and cookies at movie theaters, and a lot of other sweet temptations.

Here are some tools to beat the sugar cravings. The sooner (age wise) you realize and deal with it, the easier it is to avoid the weight gain and the diabetes.

- Avoid the usual insults. In college you are the one who shops, so remember sugary, unhealthy foods are easier not to have at home or in the dorm room.
- Do not miss a meal; three regular meals a day or five to six smaller

meals daily help to avoid the hunger attack. Add protein to each meal. Protein stretches hunger-free periods and so does fiber.

- Eating breakfast helps with carbohydrate cravings throughout the day. It's shown by several studies that missing breakfast messes up the metabolism.
- Replace empty, sugary foods with fruits. Instead of a flavored yogurt, have a plain yogurt with frozen berries. If midafternoon is the usual time for sugar craving, keep some snacks around, like nuts, a square or two of dark chocolate, cheese and crackers, carrot sticks, or a food bar.
- If the craving is unbearable, have an Altoid or chew gum. Strong cravings usually go away in several minutes. If you satisfy your sweet tooth, it comes right back and you crave more.
- Reward yourself with dark chocolate or an occasional fancy pastry. Blend fruits and nuts, freeze in the form of cubes, and eat them instead of ice cream. Ice cream that is made from cream and sugar (not high fructose corn syrup or artificial sweetener) is also okay in small amounts. Because of the fat, it shouldn't contribute to food cravings, but do it if you can eat only two scoops and not every day.

* * *

14. Slow Food nation

The term "Slow Food" was coined by Carlo Petrini, who was outraged when a McDonald's opened near the historic Spanish Steps in Rome nearly two decades ago. The Slow Food philosophy wants Americans to "vote with their fork," eat locally grown and organic food, rediscover the joys of cooking, enjoy meals with family and friends, and support local farmers. But in a nation that invented large-scale farming, fast food, and TV dinners, that's been an uphill battle.

The Slow Food movement now has 85,000 members in 132 countries and is beginning to catch on in the United States of America. It's supported by thought leaders such as Eric Schlosser, author of *Fast Food Nation*, Alice Waters, founder of Chez Panisse Restaurant in Berkeley, California, and Michael Pollan, author of *The Omnivore's Dilemma* and *In Defense of Food*.

It is apparent that slow food is the antithesis of fast food. For a taste of the slow-food concept, one may contemplate the scope of the perceived problems and challenges with our food supply. Here are some:

- Much of what is available in the form of fast food comprises cheaply made, nutrient-poor, long-lived, and calorie-dense items such as french fries, high fructose corn syrup, white buns, burgers, milkshakes, and sodas.
- People who consume these products tend to become overweight or obese. Fast-food consumers tend to have high cholesterol, diabetes, heart disease, and cancers.
- Petroleum products are heavily used in food production in the form

of fuel for farm equipment, chemicals and energy for fertilizer, pesticide production and application, transportation, packaging, and refrigeration. Food products often travel thousands of miles from farm to supermarket shelf.

- The concept of slow food is that by redesigning the modern food production and delivery system, we can improve our diets with the added benefit of reduced dependence on petroleum and stronger local economies. As an example, overcrowded factory farms in the Midwest are replaced by more traditional cattle farms spread out throughout the country as was the case not so many years ago. Open-pasture grazing means that the beef will contain less saturated fat, and there will be less reliance on antibiotics and less risk of deadly E. coli infections. The meat will probably taste better, too. But would the consumer be willing to pay the higher cost per pound of meat? After all it's all about value, or, more precisely, the price. Isn't this how we got into an epidemic of unhealthiness in the first place?

Here are some suggestions:

- As you stroll through your next farmer's market, take notice of farm produce grown in nearby communities, even within your own county.
- Stop and admire food produced organically, and compliment the growers. Buy some, too.
- When you see "fair trade" imported items such as coffee, ask the seller what that means.
- Cook yourself a meal using ingredients that you know were produced in your own state.

* * *

15. Don't buy or eat anything your great-grandmother or your grandmother wouldn't recognize as food

Don't you love looking at black and white pictures of your ancestors? Have you noticed that they are all slim (particularly at younger age)? Well, if your grandparent was overweight, then he or she might have a genetic form of obesity. But most grandparents weren't even mildly overweight, and they didn't starve either.

How do you suppose our grandparents and great-grandparents ate? Do you suppose our ancestors ate french fries? Candy? Gatorade? Diet Coke? How often do you think they ate pizza, chocolate, ice cream, white rice, or white processed bread? Do you suppose they ate meat every day? Did they drink orange juice every day? Did they eat bananas because "they're supposed to have lots of potassium"?

What happened within the last 40–50 years that changed the looks and the weight of humanity?

- Fast-food chains are serving high-fat, high-carbohydrate meals that are enjoyed universally. Working moms are saved from prolonged traditional cooking. There are no dirty dishes and kids love it.
- There is a direct correlation between the introduction of high fructose corn syrup (HFCS) into foods and the obesity epidemic that started in 1975.
- Lots of snacks are high in fat and carbohydrates and low in fiber. Many companies fill up their break rooms with candy, chips, sodas, and chocolate chip cookies. It tastes even better when it is free.

- Traditional American parties fill up with chips and dips, burgers and hot dogs, piñatas and party bags full of candy. Not to mention Halloween.
- Personal cars for everybody, escalators, elevators, remote controls.
- Computers, videos, video games.

Welcome to the Great Eating Scam. Successful marketing depends on delivery of a uniform product. And suddenly, it makes sense. Orange drink replaces orange juice. Crystal Light replaces real lemonade. Bacon has "smoky flavor" as a listed ingredient, and your toothpaste gel is a beautiful blue. Predictable. Familiar. I don't want to sound paranoid, but when I read what I wrote, I certainly do. And so does G. K. Chesterton when he claimed, "Progress is the mother of problems."

Avoid the foods that your grandma or great-grandma would not recognize, and you will avoid a variety of low-nutrient, high-calorie, and unnecessary-for-your-health foods. Your great-grandma didn't need to read labels, but you do.

* * *

16. Get off your butt

"Those who think they have no time for bodily exercise will sooner or later have to find time for illness."

Edward Stanley

One thing you do a lot in college is study, which translates to "sit" for your body and "think" for your brain. You certainly have hundreds of lazy bones under your skin, just like the rest of us. And when studying gets you tired, nothing gets you perked up like a grande-Java-chip-triple-mocha latte. A quick, full-of-calories fix! It's a jolt to the brain, and then you can go back studying. But what about the body? Hopefully, you're walking to Starbucks for 30 minutes to get yourself some venti, high-sugar, high-fat, high-calorie drink. Many, however, just walk to the refrigerator and grab a can of soda or Frappuccino, and ten steps later are sitting back at the desk. Not ignoring the needs of the body will pay off, and vice versa.

The Swedish scientists from the Karolinska Institute argue that prolonged periods of sitting are different from the term "sedentary behavior," which means a general lack of exercise. Based on their research, they suggest "muscular inactivity" is a term that more accurately describes a state of prolonged immobility, like when you sit and study for a long time or sit in front of the computer or the TV. This is important, because research shows that periods of prolonged sitting and lack of whole-body muscular activity is strongly associated with the development of diabetes, obesity, heart disease, and cancer, regardless of whether moderate or vigorous exercise was performed. This goes to show that maintaining an intermittent level of activity that involves total body muscle movement (climbing stairs, walking to run errands, taking a walking break during sedentary work) is just as important as incorporating moderate to vigorous exercise into your routine.

So even if you exercise once or twice a week but happen to spend most of your time sitting, you're still raising your own risk of all of the diseases mentioned above. Here is an action point. Once every couple of hours, take a 10–15 minute break and stretch, jump rope, run up and down the stairs, or go for a walk. Your brain, as well as your body, will feel rejuvenated when it's time for you to once again hit the books.

* * *

17. Watch out for salt

Salt has been targeted as a public enemy for many years. Its connection to hypertension (high blood pressure) is clear, but the connection to weight gain or heart disease is not as obvious. Government nutrition guidelines now call for adults to limit their daily sodium intake to less than 2,300 milligrams a day—the equivalent of about a teaspoon of table salt.

Salt has no calories, so why is it that we need to cut down on salty foods? People who consume salt and also drink lots of water are unable to lose weight for the simple reason that water has a weight and doesn't get excreted from the body in the presence of salt.

There is a funny diet called the ape diet—people eat only raw foods, nuts, fruits, vegetables and small amount of meat. Within days of starting this diet, participants lost about nine pounds of weight. Interestingly, their total calories weren't decreased—they had been given 2,000–2,500 calories of total daily food. But what changed was the sodium content, which decreased from 12 grams to 1 gram per day. Now this diet is very hard (it's not easy to be an ape), and while I don't promote that you try the ape diet, the lessons are very obvious. Raw food doesn't contain much salt, but once the food is prepared or canned, a lot of salt is snuck into it by a corporate cook. Even if you are not hypertensive and do not have metabolic syndrome, eating more than 5 grams of salt per day will hinder your weight loss by promoting fluid retention. Here are some of the salt contents in different commonly consumed foods:

1. Most cereals have about 300 milligrams per cup.
2. Vegetable juices have about 650 milligrams of salt.
3. A cup of canned cream-style corn contains 730 milligrams of sodium.
4. Beef or pork salami (2 slices) can pack 604 milligrams of sodium.
5. A cup of chicken noodle soup (canned) contains as much as 1,106 milligrams of sodium, and a cup of Nissin chicken-flavored noodles has 1,170 milligrams.
6. Teriyaki sauce (1 tablespoon) contains 690 milligrams of sodium, and soy sauce (1 tablespoon) may contain up to 1,000 milligrams of sodium.
7. Half a cup of spaghetti sauce may pack 610 milligrams of sodium—and that amount barely coats a helping of pasta.
8. Salt is in condiments—canned jalapeno peppers (¼ cup, solids and liquids) contain about 434 milligrams of sodium. Ketchup (1 tablespoon) has 178 milligrams, sweet relish (1 tablespoon) has 121milligrams, and capers (1 tablespoon) have 255 milligrams.
9. Some obvious ones, per 1-ounce serving:

   • Potato chips = 149 milligrams
   • Cheese puffs = 258 milligrams
   • Pretzels = 385 milligrams

Every ethnic food that comes to mind (Chinese, Japanese, Italian, French, Mexican, or any of the Middle Eastern cuisines) has too much salt. You can see how easy it is to get to 10–12 grams of sodium a day. Reading labels will help to sort it out, and don't forget the portion sizes. So you don't need to eliminate the salt completely, but try to stay under 5 grams per day, and less than that if you have metabolic syndrome or diabetes.

* * *

18. How to be a healthy vegetarian

A vegetarian is someone who does not eat meat, including beef, chicken, pork, or fish. Some vegetarians may or may not choose to eat animal products such as eggs, milk, gelatin, or honey. There are different types of vegetarians:

Lacto-ovo vegetarian

Lacto–ovo vegetarians do not eat meat but do eat eggs and dairy products ("ovo" means eggs and "lacto" means dairy).

Lacto vegetarian

Lacto vegetarians do not eat meat but do eat dairy products.

Ovo vegetarian

Ovo vegetarians do not eat meat but do eat eggs.

Vegan

Vegans avoid eating any animal products. Vegans do not eat any meat products, milk, cheese, eggs, honey, or gelatin. Many vegans choose not to wear clothes containing animal products, such as leather, wool, or silk, or wear makeup tested on animals

People decide to become vegetarians for many reasons. Some common motivators include the environment, animal rights, and health. You may have different reasons. Deciding to become vegetarian is an individual decision. Vegetarian diets can be very healthy, but eating a balanced diet when you are vegetarian usually requires a little extra attention. Because vegetarians eliminate certain foods from their diets, they often need to work to add foods into their diet that will provide the nutrients found in meat products. By eating a variety of foods, including fruits, vegetables, and whole grains, you can get nutrients you need from nonmeat sources. Vegans need to pay special attention to getting enough protein, iron, calcium, vitamin D, and vitamin B12.

Foods high in protein like nuts, peanut butter, soy foods, and legumes such as beans, peas, and lentils should be incorporated into daily menus. Protein is also found in dairy foods such as milk, yogurt, and cheese for vegetarians who eat these foods.

Iron is found in beans, seeds, soy foods, fortified breakfast cereals, and dark green, leafy vegetables like spinach. Vitamin C helps our body to absorb iron, so it is important to eat foods rich in vitamin C, such as citrus fruits and certain vegetables (such as tomatoes) as well.

Calcium is required to build strong bones. Calcium is found in dairy products such as milk, yogurt, and cheese. Some foods are not naturally high in calcium but have calcium added to them; these foods are called calcium fortified. Some soy products, orange juices, cereals, and cereal bars are calcium fortified. Look at the Nutrition Facts Label to find out which brands are highest in calcium. Calcium intake is important for both men and women, and for college students the adequate intake is about 1,300 mg. You don't need an actual supplement if you're taking that much from food (1 cup yogurt has 450 milligrams and 1 cup kale or other greens about 100 milligrams). Vegans will have a hard time getting that much from their food and will require supplementation. Most fortified foods contain 500 to 1,000 milligrams of calcium per serving.

Vitamin D is necessary for strong bones and has been implicated in preventing a variety of health issues. Its intake is particularly important for people who live in colder climates, because you need the sun to make your own vitamin D. During the winter, the sun is not as strong and you are not able to make enough vitamin D. Therefore, it is especially important to make sure you get vitamin D from fish and the foods you eat, such as fortified dairy products and soy milk, or from a supplement of 800 to 2000 I.U. (international units) of vitamin D daily.

Vitamin B12 is found in animal foods, so vegans must eat foods fortified with B12. Examples include nutritional yeast flakes, fortified soy milk, fortified cereals, or a supplement.

Becoming vegetarian or vegan is a major step. As long as you do your research and learn about the necessary supplements, it is a healthy diet and behavior.

* * *

19. What supplements do you need to take?

Many nutrients and vitamins are not produced by our body and should be imported with food. We need about 40 different nutrients a day to survive: that includes 14 different vitamins, eight to 10 amino acids, 15 minerals, and two fatty acids. All of those vitamins, nutrients, and minerals are available in whole foods and dairy, and can be consumed with food. However, the American Medical Association recommends taking a multivitamin daily. The reason is that most people in this country practice an American or Western lifestyle and lack some or many important nutrients.

The Recommended Dietary Allowance or RDA (sometimes referred to as Recommended Daily Allowance) is defined as "the average daily dietary intake level that is sufficient to meet the nutrient requirements of nearly all (approximately 98 percent) healthy individuals." DRI, or Dietary Reference Intake, is the newest term replacing the RDA. All this information is usually on the label of the supplements. If you are a healthy eater, consuming your daily colorful fruits and vegetables, you get all the water-soluble vitamins (B and C) and minerals from those. Those vitamins are required for the body daily and need to be consumed daily. If you do not eat daily fruits and vegetables, then taking a multivitamin is a good idea. Vitamin B12 is necessary for red blood cells, nerve functioning, and many metabolic processes. It also used to regenerate folate and thymine. It is found in red meat, liver, clams, shellfish, and in small amounts in dairy. Vegetarians, and especially vegans, will require regular B12 supplementation.

The fat-soluble vitamins A, D, K, and E are stored by the body and do not require daily consumption. Eating animal products like, meat, dairy, and fish, for an otherwise healthy person, should be enough to store and avoid deficiencies. Our bodies convert ultraviolet B rays into vitamin D. But for a variety of reasons—sunscreen, clothing, and pollution—there is a lot of vitamin D deficiency in the United States and elsewhere. It turns out that vitamin D is not just necessary for the bone strength, but it contributes to our immune system and vascular health as well.

Food sources of vitamin D are fish liver oil, the flesh of fatty fish, the fat from seals and polar bears (yummy!), and fortified milk. Unfortunately, many people do not drink enough milk and avoid eating polar bears; plus, it's not clear that even if you do consume those things, you'll get a sufficient level in the blood. So, it's obvious that we need to supplement vitamin D, but then how much and what kind? There is D3 that is naturally occurring and D2 that occurs in plants in small amounts but mostly is produced as a prescription medicine. The D3 is the one you need. The official recommendation for vitamin D is 200 to 600 I.U per day, depending on age. However, most people who take that much vitamin D still have levels below normal. While officials of the U.S. Advisory Board are waiting for more data to support increasing the recommended dosage, we suggest people take at least 1,000 I.U and up to 2,000 I.U in the winter months. It is cheap and safe, and those doses do not have any side effects.

* * *

20. Eat mindfully

Mindful eating is the opposite of mindless eating. Mindless eating is something that most people have done in some or other ways. There are many examples of mindless eating, including dieting, eating to get relief from stress, bingeing, snacking, grabbing a doughnut from a break room, having popcorn and soda at a movie theater, and many other examples of automatic or mindless eating.

Dieting is a good example: the cabbage soup diet, low-carb diets, or any other miracle diets usually end with our "falling off the wagon" and gaining even more weight. Most people trying to lose weight have tried multiple diets. Mindful eating is a part of a lifestyle, not a temporary effort.

Eating mindfully is a process. It's like martial arts. It's a skill that takes time to build. By eating mindfully, we treat our body and mind mindfully. Macrobiotic eating is a good example of mindful eating. It should not be called a diet; it's more like a conscious lifestyle. Macrobiotic eating is paying a lot of attention to the way of eating. It's not something new but a way of eating that includes more vegetarian dishes, low protein items, and foods high in whole grain.

Many of the simple recommendations that we have been talking about in our program, such as eating breakfast or eating three times per day, are examples of mindful eating. A good example of mindful eating is vegetarianism. Vegetarians give up certain foods not because they don't want meat, are allergic to it, or are on a temporary crash diet. Their reasons for abstaining from certain foods are more conceptual, religious, environmental, or healthful. They are consistent with their food relationship on a regular basis. I'm not trying to make anyone become vegetarian, but I advise you to eat just as mindfully as vegetarians do, by observing the food and making healthy choices in food every day.

Here are some recommendations for building the skill of mindful eating:

- Stay attuned to your relationship with food.
- Plan your meals and make shopping lists.
- Observe the food and learn your nutrients. Eating junk food and taking vitamins is a perfect example of mindless eating.
- Eat slowly. Get up from the table while you still have some room in your tummy.
- By eating mindfully, you support the environment. Shop at farmer's markets.
- Treat your guests the same way you treat your body. Don't buy soda just for your guests, cookies just for little sisters and brothers, or cake from Costco except for birthdays. That is mindful cheating.
- At restaurants, refuse the second serving of bread and butter. Those are shown to be the most frequent restaurant-related mindless eating examples.
- There will be setbacks, because mindless habits are strong. Don't worry if you face those sometimes.
- Taking walks and exercising is a part of the mindful treatment of the body.

It takes a while to master mindful eating. The jug fills up drop by drop. Improve your relationship with food and enjoy mindful eating.

* * *

21. Break bad eating habits

Identifying emotional eating triggers and bad eating habits is the first step; however, this alone is not sufficient to alter eating behavior. Usually, by the time you have identified a pattern, eating in response to emotions or certain situations has become a habit. Now you have to break that habit. Developing alternatives to eating is the second step. When you start to reach for food in response to an eating trigger, try one of the following activities instead.

- Read a good book or magazine, or listen to music.
- Go for a walk or jog.
- Take a bubble bath.
- Do deep breathing exercises.
- Play cards or a board game.
- Talk to a friend.
- Do housework, laundry, or yard work.
- Wash the car.
- Write a letter.
- Do any other pleasurable or necessary activity until the urge to eat passes.
- Start a new rule in your place—no food allowed in the TV room.

Sometimes simply distracting yourself from eating and developing alternative habits is not enough to manage the emotional distress that leads to excessive eating. To more effectively cope with emotional stress, try the following:

- Relaxation exercises
- Meditation
- Individual or group counseling

These techniques address the underlying emotional problems which are causing you to binge and teach you to cope in more effective and healthier ways.

As you learn to incorporate more appropriate coping strategies and to curb excessive eating, remember to reward yourself for a job well done. We tend to repeat behaviors that have been reinforced, so reward yourself when you meet your weight loss goals. Buy a new shirt, a not-too-expensive ring or earrings, or get that massage you wanted. By rewarding yourself for a job well done, you increase the likelihood that you will maintain your new healthy habits.

* * *

22. Restaurant dining

Imagine walking into a fast-food restaurant and seeing the number of calories for each item up on the overhead menu. How would that affect the way your order? A provision of the federal health care reform legislation passed in March of 2010 gives chain restaurants up to a year to begin posting nutritional information in regular items. They are also required to post information about the average number of calories consumed by a healthy person in one day.

According to the National Restaurant Association, Americans eat almost 24% of their meals at restaurants. Making poor choices when eating out, such as splurging and not paying attention to calories consumed, is a direct cause of weight gain. Armed with a little knowledge, you can put together a healthier meal at almost any restaurant without sacrificing taste and price. There are two main problems with restaurant food: portion sizes and hidden or obvious calories. Even if you order a healthy meal, most restaurants give you far too much. Fortunately, most supply takeout boxes, so you can take a doggy bag and turn tonight's dinner into tomorrow's lunch.

What about calories? In restaurants where nutritional information is not available, following a few simple rules can help you order wisely, whether you're at a local deli or sampling exotic ethnic cuisines.

- Choose meals that center on lean meats and veggie-based sauces, instead of thick and fatty cuts of meat and cream sauces.
- In a delicatessen, you have more control over your meal. Often, they give you the option to build your own sandwich, so you can

choose whole-wheat bread, rye, or pumpernickel, not just pure white bread. Beyond the bread, be careful of the meats and cheeses. Hold the salami and extra cheese, as these tend to be high in fat and sodium; opt for the low-fat turkey or even low-fat ham. Don't skimp on veggies, such as tomatoes, onions, cucumbers, peppers, avocados, or sprouts. For condiments, skip the mayo and go for mustard or a small amount of hummus, bean paste, and/or pepper for spice.

- Unlike authentic Chinese food, the heavily Americanized Chinese food we know is usually served with fried rice and sugary sauces. Avoid these high-sugar, low-substance foods whenever possible. Unfortunately, that includes a good chunk of the menu at many Chinese restaurants, including favorites like egg rolls, fried shrimp or meat, spare ribs, ad infinitum. Also, watch out for foods on the Chinese menu that tend to be dripping in sauces, like the sweet-and-sour chicken or pork. Go for the nonfried chicken, or options that are heavy on the veggies and light on the sauce, like brown rice with vegetables. Boiled, steamed, or lightly stir-fried seafood, chicken, vegetables, or bean curd dishes are generally low in fat but are hidden on the menus. At any Chinese fast-food place, you can order steamed green beans, cauliflower, and broccoli. Even those who don't list low-cal dishes on the menu are often willing to steam a dish instead of frying and make other modifications.
- American Italian restaurants offer up some tasty options for people watching their diets. Stay away from pastas stuffed with cheese or meat, as well as dishes topped with cheese. Keep in mind that "parmigiana style" usually translates into higher fat. Choose pasta with marinara sauce (tomato based) instead of creamy white or butter sauces, such as Alfredo. If you are in the mood for pizza, portion control is the key. Start with a salad. Ask for thin crust, vegetables, extra marinara sauce, and half the cheese.
- In Mexican restaurants choose dishes made with plain, soft tortillas that aren't fried, like burritos or enchiladas. Pick baked entrees, corn tortillas, and Mexican rice. Use salsa instead of sour cream or cheese dips. Go easy on the corn chips.

- All-American food like hamburgers, onion rings, buffalo wings, and french fries are usually very heavy in calories. But there are better choices, like barbecued chicken or grilled chicken, pot roast, meat loaf with tomato sauce, filet mignon or sirloin steak, or a turkey pita sandwich. Pita sandwiches have become more popular, and the whole-wheat variety is an excellent choice. Soups with beans and lentils are a great choice, while clam chowder is very heavy. When ordering a salad, always ask for the dressings on the side, and use a quarter of the portion you're given. Ask for grilled or steamed veggies instead of fried. The waiters are used to it by now and are happy to assist you.
- If you absolutely have to order dessert, share it with your friends. Not to spoil your appetite, but a typical apple pie slice served at Marie Callender's has 860 calories. Dining out is supposed to be a pleasant experience. Enjoy healthy dining!

* * *

23. Summary of the action points of the Alpha Plan

- Know your nutrition facts, educate yourself about health, and learn how to prevent common medical problems earlier in life.
- Make exercise a priority in daily life.
- Know what to shop for. Make a list, avoiding processed and packaged foods.
- Limit TV and computer use to a minimum. This is the hardest.
- Sleep eight hours every night.
- Drink plenty of water.
- Drink coffee and tea without adding any sweeteners. Avoid soft drinks and limit fruit juice.
- Know the consequences of excessive alcohol use.
- Eat plenty of vegetables and fruits. Try new vegetables.
- Eat breakfast daily. Eat lean protein to control appetite.
- Eat whole grains. Eat a variety of foods.
- Learn to cook and enjoy cooking healthy meals.
- Eat mindfully.
- Learn your stress triggers and how to avoid them.
- Avoid fast food and soft drinks.
- Remember that you can eat anything you want, as long as you are careful about what you want!

* * *

Bibliography

Bell, R., et al. Correlates of college student marijuana use: results of a U.S. National Survey. *Addiction*. 1997 May; 92(5):571-81.

Bowe, W. P., et al. Diet and acne. *J Am Acad Dermatol*. 2010 Jul; 63(1):124-41. Epub 2010 Mar

Brousseau, M. E., and E. J. Schaefer. Diet and coronary heart disease: clinical trials. *Curr Atheroscler Rep*. 2000; 2:487–49.

Burke, G. L., et al., Artery Risk Differences in weight gain in relation to race, gender, age and education in young adults: the CARDIA Study. Coronary Development in Young Adults. *Ethn Health*. 1996 Dec; 1(4):327-35.

Ford, E. S., et al. "Trends in the Prevalence of Low Risk Factor Burden for Cardiovascular Disease Among United States Adults." *Circulation*, 2009.

Foster, G. D., et al. "Weight and metabolic outcomes after 2 years on a low-carbohydrate versus low-fat diet: A randomized trial." *Ann Intern Med* 2010; 153:147-157.

Gearhardt, A. N., et al. "Neural correlates of food addiction." *Arch Gen Psych* 2011; DOI: 10.1001/archgenpsychiatry.2011.32.

Harris, J., et al. "Effects of serving high-sugar cereals on children's breakfast-eating behavior." *Pediatrics* 2011; 127:71-76.

Hull, Holly R., et al. The effect of the Thanksgiving Holiday on weight gain *Nutr J*. 2006; 5:29.

Hood, E. Organic Food for Thought: Lessening Children's Pesticide Exposure. *Environ Health Perspect*, 2003. 111:a166-a166. doi:10.1289/ehp.111-a166a.

Kistler, K. D., et al. Physical activity recommendations, exercise intensity, and histological severity of nonalcoholic Fatty liver disease. *Am J Gastroenterol*. 2011 Mar; 106(3):460-8.

Kolotkin, Ronette L., et al., Obesity and Sexual Quality of Life, *Obesity* (2006) 14, 472–479; 10.1038/oby.2006.62.

Leproult, Rachel, et al.; Role of Sleep and Sleep Loss in Hormonal Release and Metabolism, *Endocr Dev*. 2010; 17:11–21.

Liu, Y., et al. Food addiction and obesity: evidence from bench to bedside; *J Psychoactive Drugs*. 2010 Jun; 42(2):133-45.

Malik, V. S., et al. Popular weight-loss diets: from evidence to practice. *Nat Clin Pract Cardiovasc Med*. 2007; 4:34–36.

Myers, J., R. Arena, B. Franklin, I. Pina, W. E. Kraus, K. McInnis, and G. J. Balady. American Heart Association Committee on Exercise, Cardiac Rehabilitation, and Prevention of the Council on Clinical Cardiology, the Council on Nutrition, Physical Activity, and Metabolism, and the Council on Cardiovascular Nursing. *Circulation*. 2009 Jun 23; 119(24):3144-61.

Nestle, Marion. *Food Politics*.University of California Press, Berkley and Los Angeles, 2007.

Parks, E. J., et al. "Dietary sugars stimulate fatty acid synthesis in adults." *J Nutr* 2008; 138:1039-1046.

Patel, Raj. *The Value of Nothing*.Picador, New York, 2009.

Pollan, Michael. *The Omnivore's Dilemma*. Penguin Press, New York, 2006.

Rundle, Andrew, et al. Neighborhood Food Environment and Walkability Predict Obesity in New York City. *Environmental Health Perspectives*. 2009; 117(3):442-447.

Sacks, Frank M., et al. Comparison of Weight-Loss Diets with Different Compositions of Fat, Protein, and Carbohydrates, *N Engl J Med* 2009; 360:859-873, February 26, 2009.

Schlosser, Eric. *Fast Food Nation*, Harper Collins, New York, 2001.

Stranges, et al. Cross-sectional versus Prospective Associations of Sleep Duration with Changes in Relative Weight and Body Fat Distribution: The Whitehall II Study. *American Journal of Epidemiology*. 2008; 167(3):321-32923.

Suzuki, K., K. A. Simpson, J. S. Minnion, J. C. Shillito, and S. R. Bloom. The role of gut hormones and the hypothalamus in appetite regulation. *Endocr J*. 2010; 57(5):359-72.

Vasanti, S., Malik, Sugar Sweetened Beverages, Obesity, Type 2 Diabetes and Cardiovascular Disease risk. *Circulation*. 2010 March 23; 121(11):1356–1364.

Web Sites

http://www.medscape.com
http://www.medpagetoday.com
http://www.collegedrinkingprevention.gov/NIAAACollegeMaterials
http://choosemyplate.gov
http://www.localharvest.org
http://www.diabetes.org
http://Wikipedia.org

Part 3.
Eating in College

1. Dorm living and no-stove eating

Moving into a dorm and being away from home for the first time is a huge thrill. You get to meet tons of new people, plunge yourself into a new academic life, and basically learn how to survive on your own. Sometimes, though, there are hidden stresses involved in such a huge change in your life. In addition to learning in class, you will have to actually think about meal planning, exercise, and fitness for fitness' sake, sleep, and overall health because there is no one else to do it for you anymore. Welcome to an adult world.

This chapter is designed to help you navigate through dorm living without a stove, and then on to apartment living with a real kitchen.

What foods should you keep in the dorm room?

Face it, you will get hungry in your dorm room during off hours when the dining hall is closed or when it is too hot or cold to walk over to it. Breakfast is often missed because you are running late to class and can't make the time to stop and eat. What can you do to be prepared for when that happens?

Every dorm room these days has a small microwave, small refrigerator, and either a small coffee maker or hot water heater which is provided by the students. With this in mind, you can easily prepare simple foods for those times when you can't get over to the dining hall.

Many collegiates think that they don't have enough time in the morning to sit down and eat a meal. If you're running short on time, remember that any meal is better than no meal at all. Plan on keeping certain foods on hand in your dorm refrigerator that you can eat when getting ready for school or work such as:

- Yogurts
- Small cartons of milk or soy milk
- Cheese sticks
- Hard-boiled eggs (from the dining hall)
  On one of your shelves you can keep easy-to-eat foods such as:
- Granola bars
- Fruit
- Small boxes of cereal or packets of oatmeal
- Trail mix or nuts
- Bread for sandwiches
- Peanut butter or other nut butter
- Honey and jam
- Instant coffee or tea bags
- Energy bars, like Clif, Luna, Balance, Odwalla, etc.
  Fresh water

* * *

2. Breakfast

"Eat your breakfast, share your lunch with a friend, and give your dinner to the enemy," says the old Russian proverb, hyperbolically, but the message is obvious. Rushing to school or other activities often makes eating breakfast a challenge. There are lots of benefits to eating a healthy breakfast, such as having more energy to perform your best at school and in sports. This guide will give you breakfast ideas so you can start your day off right and have energy that will last all morning—no more falling asleep in class! Research has shown that people who eat breakfast regularly:

- Do better in school than those who don't, and have a better attention span;
- Are less likely to be overweight than those who skip breakfast;
- Are more likely to meet their daily vitamin and mineral needs;
- Eat more fiber and calcium and less fat than people who skip breakfast.

Eating breakfast in the dining hall

When choosing a healthy breakfast, aim for a protein to start your day and build around that. Fiber and protein are the most filling nutrients, so if you tend to get hungry in the morning, be sure to include protein-rich foods and fiber-rich foods. Protein-rich foods include eggs, peanut or other nut butters, nuts, soy products, milk, yogurt, meats, and cheese. Fiber-rich foods include fruits, vegetables, and whole grains. For example, a bowl of oatmeal with nuts and fruit will keep you full much longer than a bowl of sugary cereal or a dough-nut. The sweet breakfasts will make you crash in a few hours and you won't be able to stay awake in class or on the job. Below are a few healthy breakfast ideas that can come from either a dining hall or your dorm room.

Breakfast Parfait	1 cup whole-grain cold cereal mixed with yogurt and topped with fruit, such as bananas or berries (use seasonal fruit, which is the freshest and usually the cheapest if you are on your own); water, coffee, or tea
Fast and Simple	A cheese stick or hard-boiled egg, a seasonal piece of fruit, and a granola bar; water, coffee, or tea
Hot Cereal	Microwave hot oatmeal or Zoom (wheat cereal) with low-fat milk and topped with fresh fruit and/or nuts; water, coffee, or tea

Also, take a look at dining hall nutritional guides. They are usu-ally posted online. Remember, protein, fiber (fruit or vegetable), and grain: PB&J on whole-grain bread with a side of banana or apple; or, English muffin with a poached egg and tomato, and fruit on the side. Make your own meals based on the basics. If you have time, sit down and eat. You will love your body and yourself when you take good care of you. If you have to run, grab an energy bar, a cup of coffee or tea, or a glass of OJ.

3. Snack foods in the dorm room

Aside from regular meals, you may want to snack in your room. The reality is you will get hungry in your room when there is no place to go for food or beverage. Hence, the need for a basic supply of nibbles to hold you over until the dining hall opens up. Besides cookies, chips, and Cokes, which we hope you will limit, there are other great-tasting foods that will satisfy your hunger and will keep well on your shelves and in your dorm fridge. Keep your snacks simple. You don't need to spend a lot of time preparing your own dorm room foods, but you do need to think ahead. Some suggestions for good snacks include:

- Hummus and pita chips
- Salsa and baked tortilla chips
- Cereal and milk
- Energy bars
- Fruits and veggies (carrot and celery sticks, apples, cutie Clementine tangerines, bananas, or other fruits picked up from the dining hall)
- Almonds or nut mixes (go for the raw unsalted kind)
- Peanut or other nut butters, whole-wheat bread, and jam for peanut butter and jelly sandwiches
- Top Ramen or other instant noodle meals

One of the hardest things is not to snack on junk food. Even if you don't keep junk food in your room, other people in the dorms will. There are stories of kids eating whole large bags of chips in one sitting while socializing or watching TV in the rooms. The salt, sugars, and fat taste really good and will satisfy you for about 10 minutes. The reality is that the whole bag of chips will make you feel gross sooner or later. There is so much fat and salt combined with no nutrition that your brain actually feels clogged.

Limit the junk food and stick with those healthier choices, and after a while you won't even crave bad snacks anymore.

* * *

4. Dorm food nutritional guides

This advertisement comes from a nationally ranked college. Clearly its efforts are well-intentioned, but you worked hard to get here, so why do you have to fight the food?

"College" Buffet

You will have more time to study and socialize while you live at "College." Avoid the inconvenience of cooking and the expense of grocery shopping. "College" buffet offers a variety of meal plans to suit your schedule and budget. The food is prepared fresh daily, nutritious, delicious, and always "all you can eat!"

Choose from three different meal plans: 7, 10, or 14 meals per week, served in our scenic creekside dining room. Make your own sandwich at the deli bar, create your own salad at the salad bar, and enjoy a variety of entrees, drinks, and desserts. Going to be at school all day? Take a sack lunch to school with you. Check out this week's buffet menu at "College"...

It is a gift to be able to pick up any food you want and prepare foods to go if you are going to be in class during a meal time. As with any restaurant, there are bonuses and pitfalls. Learning how to navigate your choices will benefit you in the long run.

Start with drinks: a large portion of drinks offered are sodas or other artificially sweetened or flavored beverages. Milks and waters are available but sometimes are not as prominently displayed. If you like ice tea, make sure it doesn't have high fructose corn syrup or artificial sweetener in it. Try to learn to drink ice tea with just lemon. If you like juice, make sure that it is just that, fruit juice, and that it doesn't have added sugar or artificial sweeteners (such as aspartame, sucralose, or saccharin).

Starchy foods are often used as fillers in most buffets. They are an inexpensive way to offer large portions and keep the cost down for the cafeteria or restaurant. A typical example is mashed potatoes or white pasta. A serving size for any of the starches is ½–1 cup. Learn how to serve yourself or ask for less and then take advantage of more variety of foods on your plate. Be careful about what you are served at the pasta bar. Some of the portions are about three times as much as a person should eat in one sitting! Tell the servers how much you want—they will listen.

Why do you need an all-you-can-eat buffet for every meal anyway? Are you on a cruise? This is just plain crazy. There are some very easy strategies to help you with food choices in these all-you-can-eat buffets. The same buffet will be there every day. If you don't get to eat something today, it will most likely be there tomorrow or another day, so don't feel like you need to overfill your plate if you like something.

- Pick one serving of a really good-looking protein: chicken, fish, beef, tofu, or other soy product. This should be one-fourth of your plate.
- Then pick one grain or starch: brown rice, potato, whole-grain pasta, or a bean dish. This should comprise another fourth of your plate.
- Fill the rest of your plate with salad, vegetables (more than one), and fruit.
- Save the cream sauces for no more than one time per week.
- Venture to try new types of produce. Fruits and vegetables fall into this category. A fruit salad with dinner is great in that it also helps solve the sugar cravings that oftentimes hit people later.
- Have a large glass of milk, still water, tea, or sparkling water.

If you want to select a high-fat meal, save it for one day per week. For example, after eating wisely all week, make Saturday morning your day to splurge on a huge brunch. Then take the time to go on a long walk in the afternoon or participate in some other exercise. Or if you know you have a big evening with friends or a date coming up, eat carefully for a couple days before that so that you can allow yourself an extra treat that night. Avoid all kinds of sodas. Colas contain all the bad ingredients that are making our society fat. Diet soda is just as bad for you as regular! Have you ever noticed in an airport who is drinking the diet sodas? The overweight people.

Most colleges use the Internet to post their menus for the week as well as a nutritional breakdown for them. Look at the ingredient labels on the dorm food and make sure there are no "bad" components. Remember; don't ingest high fructose corn syrup, partially hydrogenated fats, or artificial sweeteners, flavorings, or colorings. Next, look at the nutritional breakdown of protein, fat, carbohydrates, and fiber. Pay attention to the types of carbs and fats as noted in Part 1 of this book. Pick the lean protein, whole grains, and foods that are associated with good fats.

* * *

5. Care packages from the colleges

For those stressful times during finals, universities offer care packages that parents can purchase and have sent to their students. What a thoughtful idea! The parents are thinking of their kids, and the kids don't have to worry about where to get snacks. But be careful! A lot of the foods in those packages contain not-so-great food choices. You really don't want to have an energy low during a final!

Care packages come in healthy and nonhealthy varieties. The nonhealthy packages come with bags of fried and salty chips, packaged crackers with Cheez Whiz, lots of candy, salted and candied nuts, and toys. These foods leave your brain feeling unsatisfied nutritionally. The healthy packages include baked chips, cookies without artificial ingredients, soups, protein or energy bars, popcorn, coffee, and teas.

When you are worried about finals, junk food sounds delicious. However, don't overdo it with junk food just prior to taking an exam, because your brain may become nutritionally starved and your mental and physical endurance will wane.

Homemade cookies are usually fine to eat because they are made with real ingredients and aren't packaged and processed. It is hard to keep these around long because they are so good! During midterms and finals, stock fruit and veggies in the fridge along with milk, coffee, or tea. Stick to the nonfried variety of chips and snacks, avoid super-sugary foods, and remember to drink lots of water.

* * *

6. Apartment living with a kitchen

Some students have no desire to make food for themselves when all they have to do is "drive through." Granted, it will happen now and then, but this should never become a habit.

Here are some key points to plan around. Think about:

- Where you are going to eat for lunch.
- Who is available to dine with you.
- How much money you have on you and what you can afford to buy for your meal.
- How much food costs. Do you want to run up credit card debt just so you can dine out?
- What is in the vending machines and where they are located?

Eating out will add up financially and physically. Fast food and vending machines have made healthy eating that much harder in that one can get a quick fix for hunger immediately. Usually though, an unhealthy choice leads to more hunger later. Planning ahead always helps, but just the concept of planning a meal is novel for many students—first, because food was available at home and was planned by a parent, and second, because deciding what to eat is a matter of the moment.

Learning how to plan for your meals and healthy eating has a learning curve up front, but after that it becomes a no-brainer. Hang in there; menu planning and stocking your kitchen will become automatic after a while.

* * *

7. Equipping your kitchen

Most apartments and rental housing come equipped with a refrigerator, a stove, and an oven unit, and, if you are lucky, a dishwasher. Aside from that, it will be up to you to provide the rest. Two items you may want to consider purchasing, if you haven't already done so, are a blender or a small food processor (the Cuisinart brand is about $30) and a toaster, preferably a toaster oven.

Although cost is usually the biggest issue for establishing your new home, it is worth it to make certain purchases up front. For example, buying a set of dishes will save money and hassle over paper or plastic products in the long run. Ask relatives for hand-me-down items. Check out Goodwill for your kitchen needs. If you have access to a Target, Cost Plus, or Walmart, they are great places to shop for most of the items below. You can also hand the following list to your parents.

Basic dining needs:

- A place to sit, either a dining table with chairs or a counter with stools
- Dinner plates (for more durability, go with a thicker style)
- Salad plates
- Bowls for cereal and soup
- Mugs for hot drinks
- Water glasses
- Silverware: forks, knives, spoons, steak knives

Basic cooking items:

Start with the most essential items and work up from there. If you only have room or money enough for one skillet, then choose the size you want.

- Two nonstick skillets, one small one and one larger one. The smaller skillet will work well for cooking eggs, while the larger one is great for cooking main-course dishes.
- Saucepan with a lid for cooking rice, soups, stews, and steaming veggies.
- Steamer basket (make sure it fits into the saucepan).
- Large cooking pot, 5 or 6 quarts, for cooking pasta.
- Baking dish, 9x13 inches, Pyrex style, for lasagna and baked goods.
- Baking dish, either 8x8 inches or 9x9 inches, great for cooking smaller baked goods and single-serving meals.
- Cookie sheet with a small rim for baking and roasting vegetables (optional).
- Bowls: large mixing bowl, salad bowl, small bowl. Pyrex-type bowl sets are readily available, are inexpensive, and can be used for cooking, serving and storing.
- Colander for draining.
- Cutting board (get one that you can put in your dishwasher to steril- ize) and a second wooden one to cut bread on.

Cooking utensils as follows:

- Wooden spoons for stirring (two or three)
- Can opener
- Spatula for removing cookies from a baking sheet, flipping pan- cakes, serving pie or quiche, etc.
- Tongs, great for picking up food from a grill or serving
- Ladle for serving soups and stews
- Salad servers
- Measuring spoons
- Vegetable peeler
- Grater

- Kitchen knives: There are two kinds of knives that you need to know about. One is the smooth-edge blade used for slicing meats and just about everything else. The other is a serrated blade (the kind with curved teeth), which cuts bread well. Serrated blades can also be multitasking, but be aware that serrated knives often tear meat, so use a smooth-edge blade for that. You will need a small paring knife, a larger utility knife, a large serrated knife, and possibly a butcher's knife. Knife sets are quite varied in price, but just start with a basic one and work up from there.

Other kitchen necessities:

- Foil
- Plastic wrap (for storage only, never microwave plastic wrap)
- Sandwich baggies (the wax-paper brand is environmentally friendly)
- Larger storage bags (for freezer and refrigerator)
- Storage containers (some food products, such as lunch meats, come in reusable plastic containers—just don't microwave food in them)
- Liquid dish soap
- Dishwasher soap
- Dish towels (three or four)
- Oven mitts
- Paper towels
- Napkins

* * *

8. Food pantry essentials

Everyone needs a basic assortment of food items to get them started. Think about what you like to eat. If you like cereal and milk in the morning, you need to store cereal in the pantry and milk in the fridge. If you like peanut butter and jelly sandwiches, then add in good quality bread, peanut butter with no partially hydrogenated fats, and good old-fashioned jelly to your grocery list. If you like burgers for dinner, add hamburger meat, buns, lettuce, tomato, ketchup, and mustard to your list. You get the idea. The following suggested food items will work for any start-up kitchen.

- Olive oil, canola oil
- Vinegar; apple cider or balsamic vinegar is fine
- Spices: salt, pepper, garlic powder, dried thyme, dried basil, dried ginger, chili powder (this list will grow as you become accustomed to your new kitchen)
- Cereal: find high protein and high fiber varieties.
- Sugar
- Flour
- Onions
- Potatoes
- Canned goods: beans, soups and stews, tomato sauce, chopped tomatoes in juice
- Spaghetti sauce
- Pasta (try some whole-grain versions)
- Brown rice

- Salad dressing (if you are not making fresh, make sure what you buy has no artificial coloring, artificial flavoring/sweeteners, MSG, or any oils that are partially hydrogenated)
- Coffee and tea
- In-season fruits and vegetables

* * *

9. How to shop for groceries

A very simple layout is shared by every grocery store, if you can believe that. All fresh items are on the edges of the store aisles. That is where you will find your vegetables and fruits (and flowers), fresh dairy products such as milk and cheese, meat and deli counters, and bakery. Stores are designed this way for easy access to those products, which are not usually processed.

What is in the middle of the store then? It is all the packaged foods which can sit on shelves for a long time. Packaged dry foods such as cereals, pastas and grains, sauces, canned foods such as soups and beans, alcohol, sodas and other juice-type drinks, baking items and syrups, paper products, and personal items make up the inside of the store. This is where you may stumble with shopping. Label wisdom for processed dry foods will be your best asset when it comes to this part of your grocery list. On the inside shopping area of the store, you will notice that most of the food products (except for things like dried beans and rice) have long ingredient lists. On the outside edge of the store, there are rarely ingredient lists. There are no bad ingredients in a fresh head of lettuce or a bag of apples. You will be shopping in both sections, but the middle part you will need once or twice a month, whereas the perimeter shopping should be done on a weekly basis.

Making a grocery list

Every week you eat 21 meals. Seven breakfasts, seven lunches, and seven dinners. And, maybe you have some snacking in there, too.

133

How do you keep this simple? You need to ask yourself what you like to eat and how much time you are willing to spend on food preparation, planning your menu for the week, and shopping for the groceries. Also, figure in how many times a week you go out to eat. Once you have a general idea of how many meals you need to make, you can start to think about how to plan your food for the week.

For simplicity's sake, say your favorite breakfast is cereal and milk. Nutritionally you should add a piece of fruit, too. So, on your grocery list you write cereal, milk, and fruit (apples, etc.). Lunch could be a sack lunch. If you are at school or work, packing a sandwich, piece of fruit, snack pack of trail mix, and bottled water gives you more freedom to focus on your work rather than taking time away to find something to eat.

Dinners typically vary from night to night, and you probably don't want to eat the same thing over and over again. Going back to simplicity, here is an example of seven dinners:

Monday: Canned soup, grilled cheese sandwich, green salad, milk, or water.

Tuesday: Turkey burger on a whole-grain bun with lettuce, tomato, ketchup, and mustard, tossed green salad, frozen french fries, milk, or water. Use leftover ground turkey for tomorrow night's burrito if you like.

Wednesday: Vegetable or meat burrito filled with cheese, avocado, onions, tomatoes, refried beans, ground beef or turkey (optional), lettuce, rice (optional), sour cream (optional), milk or water, fruit salad.

Thursday: Baked chicken breast, green salad, baked potatoes, milk, or water.

Friday: Quesadilla filled with cheese, chicken (left over from the night before), steamed or raw vegetables, green salad, milk, or water.

Saturday: Spaghetti with meat sauce, parmesan cheese, green salad, milk, or water.

Sunday: Shrimp or chicken stir-fry with vegetables over rice or noodles, milk or water, and fruit.

Once you have your meals planned, make your grocery list. Make sure your list has proteins like chicken, fish, beef, lamb, pork, soy products, milk items, eggs, and cheese. If you are vegetarian or vegan, make sure you get foods high in protein, like legumes, tofu, seitan, nuts, and seeds. Buy those proteins which are freshest and freeze those which you don't use right away for another time. On busy days, you can make a good meal by taking advantage of prebaked or grilled chickens, premade roast meats, or the deli sections of the markets. When buying your greens, vegetables, and fruits, make sure that the produce is seasonal, preferably grown in the United States, or better locally.

Look at labels for the food products in the middle section of the grocery store. When buying canned and dry soups and stews, seasoning packets, salad dressing, sauces (barbecue, spaghetti, etc.), and ketchup, watch for high fructose corn syrup, partially hydrogenated fats, artificial sweeteners, and MSG, and don't purchase foods that contain the bad ingredients.

Avoid regular or diet sodas; try the flavored mineral waters, natural lemonades, and unsweetened teas. Real fruit juices are also good in limited amounts. Avoid or limit frappaccino-style coffees and teas loaded with artificial sweeteners, sugar, and fats.

Soup bars are also terrific but can be loaded with hidden fats and salt. Your best bets are broth-based soups with beans, lean meats, and vegetables.

Sushi from the store is fine. See if you can find brown rice sushi—it doesn't taste differently with all the seafood and veggies rolled up. Be sure you check expiration dates.

In Part 4 we have recipes and menus designed to be fairly simple and fast to make. There are a few exceptions of recipes with more complicated prep, but most of these are easy to prepare. In addition, we have considered lower fat, higher fiber, and natural ingredients in the menus that will keep your brain sharp. Most of all, be adventurous and enjoy your kitchen time.

* * *

Menu Plan and Shopping for a Week

PB&J on toast, fruit, coffee/tea	sandwich, fruit, beverage, snack	baked chicken, rice, salad, beverage
cereal and milk, fruit, coffee/tea	soup or chili, roll, snack, beverage	burrito with leftover chicken, salad, beverage
PB&J on toast, fruit, coffee/tea	sandwich, fruit, beverage, snack	turkey or beef burger, fries, salad, beverage
cereal and milk, fruit, coffee/tea	soup or chili, roll, snack, beverage	tacos with seasoned meat, salad, beans, beverage
PB&J on toast, fruit, coffee/tea	sandwich, fruit, beverage, snack	spaghetti, big salad, beverage
scrambled eggs with salsa, toast	quesadilla, fruit, beverage, snack	leftover spaghetti
cheese omelet, fruit, coffee/tea	tuna melt, salad or fruit, beverage	takeout pizza, salad, beverage

whole-grain bread for breakfast and lunch	bubbly waters	chicken breast, enough for two dinners
peanut butter	lunch meat	lettuces
Jelly	canned chili	rice
coffee or tea	rolls	broccoli
apples for breakfast and lunch	canned water-packed tuna	tortillas
bananas for breakfast and lunch	box of mac and cheese	lean ground beef
tangerines for breakfast and lunch	canned soups	taco seasoning
Milk	salad dressing or stuff to make	avocado for burrito and salads
Eggs	homemade	sour cream
cheese for breakfast, lunch, and dinner	check condiments: ketchup,	canned beans: black, pinquitos, etc.
Salsa	mustard, hot sauce	ground turkey meat
Cereal		hamburger rolls
		tomatoes
		frozen french fries
		pasta
		spaghetti sauce
		Parmesan cheese
		takeout pizza

Menu Plan and Shopping List

Mon	
Tue	
Wed	
Thu	
Fri	
Sat	
Sun	

Shopping list:

10. Cooking and eating on a budget

Buy local and fresh. Good restaurants use this technique to make the most flavorful foods at a low cost so they can make the most profit. Use this philosophy in your own kitchen. If you buy fresh produce that is in season, you can cook it simply. With older produce or foods not in season, you end up using lots of extra seasonings or sauce to mask or enhance the flavors of the not-so-flavorful foods.

    Get to know your farmer's market or local produce stands. Oftentimes, universities or companies have their own on-site stores which feature local food items. Price them out to see if they are lower in cost; you might be surprised when they are. Also, if you can buy food items close to where you are at school or work, it saves you time and the cost of gasoline.

    Get to know your seasonings. Your best allies in the kitchen will be good old salt and pepper. Also, you may want to invest in a good-quality olive oil. The basics of simple cooking usually involve these three items. Additionally, garlic powder or fresh garlic, dried or fresh ginger, dried herbs such as thyme and basil, chili powder, and various types of onions are a great way to expand your seasoning base.

    Learn how to cook cheaper cuts of meat. A whole chicken is usually a lot cheaper than cut-up chicken or just chicken breasts. A beef roast is less expensive than a steak. If you are planning on spending an evening in your apartment, allow yourself the time it takes to roast meats. A Crock-Pot or stew pot is a great fixture for cooking these kinds of proteins. And, with leftovers, future meals are taken care of.

Beans and lentils are very inexpensive and easy to use in recipes. You certainly can save money by cooking dried beans. A pound of white or black beans costs about a dollar, can be cooked in a couple of hours, and is good for several days' worth of meals and side dishes. However, canned beans are also inexpensive: you can find 15-ounce cans for under $1. Canned beans may be used in burritos, as side dishes, for soups, mixed with rice, and in bean salads. Also, they are great for serving crowds.

11 Inexpensive Foods You Should Know About:

1. Potatoes—they are filling and can be used as a side dish or part of a main dish.
2. Rice—brown rice has more fiber and protein than white.
3. Pasta and noodles—seems like every culture eats some sort of noodles.
4. Chicken—buying a whole chicken and roasting or baking it saves money over the packages that sell just breasts or thighs.
5. Beans—canned beans are an inexpensive source or protein and fiber.
6. Apples—filling and act as a quick pick-me-up during the day.
7. Canned tuna—go for the water-packed variety if you can.
8. Eggs—can be used for any meal, and contains full gamut of amino acids.
9. Cheese—a variety of types are available and add flavor, protein, and calcium.
10. Lean steak—flank steak and top round steaks are great when used with marinades and thinly sliced. Of course, try to find items on sale or buy in bulk with your friends.
11. Tofu— a consummate rescue food because you can crumble the firm type into spaghetti sauce, marinate and grill it, or blend the soft types into smoothies. Organic brands are also quite inexpensive.

* * *

Part 4.
College Cooking Made Easy
and Healthy

"Food should be fun."

Thomas Keller, chef of the French Laundry Restaurant

Many students avoid cooking for a variety of reasons: it's a mother's job, it's too complicated, there isn't enough time, they don't have the skill, and, of course, it's easier to grab cheap and delicious premade food. This part of the book is designed to assure you that all of those are myths and not facts. Simple cooking is easy and accessible to anyone. In the time it takes to deliver a greasy and low-quality pizza, you can make your own for a fraction of the cost and control exactly what goes into it, too.

As you prepare to cook a recipe, be sure to read the recipe all the way through first. Assemble all the ingredients you will need and make sure they are washed and trimmed. With some of the recipes, all you will need to do is open a can or a jar. Others may include a little more work up front, but the end result will be good. This book of recipes is for beginners and for those who want to make homey and uncomplicated recipes. The cooking time for most of our recipes is under 30 minutes for dinner and 5–10 minutes for breakfasts and lunches. The food you make has to be quick, inexpensive, and tasty for you to cook again. You should certainly venture and try more sophisticated recipes from the abundance of cookbooks and websites available.

Cleaning: Sometimes the biggest challenge for any cook, veteran or a debutant, is the cleaning part after cooking. Cooking is creative and fun, but cleaning can be hideous and tedious. Here are some tips to avoid a big mess that will deter you from future attempts to cook.

- Before starting to cook, make sure that your sink is empty and countertop is clean.
- Have a little plate/dish next to the stove to put your dirty utensils, cooking spoons, or forks on top of.
- Whatever has been used already, rinse and put into the dishwasher right away. Cutting boards, if not made out of wood, should go into the dishwasher as well. If made of wood, wash those with soap and warm water.
- If the pans and pots need to be soaked, add the hot water and leave them on the stove until you're done with all the other dishes.
- Keep a countertop spray (Mrs. Meyer's brand or any other environmentally healthy brand) handy to finish up the cleaning job.
- If you're having a party, make sure that some of the guests are in charge of cleaning.
- Clean up the mess immediately. The longer it sits, the harder the cleanup work is.

Nutritional content: We decided against reporting the nutritional content and calories for all of the recipes. It's done in many cookbooks, but we found it not crucial for this book. Food is texture and taste, not calories and nutritional components. In Parts 1 and 2 you were presented with an extensive discussion on nutrition and calories. All of our recipes are healthy and contain a normal fat and normal carbohydrate content. Actually, they are low fat and low carbohydrate if you compare them to the typical Western diet or restaurant food. If you're trying to lose weight with the help of this book, you can try every single one of the recipes.

"When baking, follow directions. When cooking, go by your own taste."

Laiko Bahrs

Follow this basic rule: When you bake, you need to follow the recipe closely (unless you are cutting down the amount of sugar you are using). But when you make breakfast, a sandwich, soup, or pasta, and you happen to be missing an ingredient, don't worry; replace it with whatever makes sense or omit it all together (as long as it's not the most important ingredient). Most importantly, remember that cooking is fun and sexy!

* * *

1. Breakfast

"Why, sometimes I've believed as many as six impossible things before breakfast."

Lewis Carroll

Always, always start your day with something to eat. Breakfast literally means to break your fast of not eating since the evening before. To make a pun, some students think that breakfast means to break, fast. Before you head off to school or work, be sure to treat yourself to food that will hold you over with protein, good carbohydrates, fiber, and essential nutrients. These elements should keep you humming until lunch time. For some, though, this will be a new habit. If you must, even a protein bar and a piece of fruit will work. Try to stick with seasonal fruit, and if not, there is always a banana. Dried fruit is available year round. Feel free to use raisins, dried cranberries, and others in your hot or cold cereals. Juices are full of sugar, natural or added. It is wiser to eat a piece of fruit and not drink fruit juice. Whole fruit is more filling and has more nutrients and fiber. However, it is okay to drink a glass of juice, use it in recipes or before workouts, and make a smoothie—just don't drink it all the time.

It is always preferable to eat your meals at the dining table, but if that is a breaking point for your breakfast, just eat something, even if it is on the run.

***

Your Favorite Cereal with Milk, Nuts, and Fruits

Make sure the cereal does not contain partially hydrogenated oils, food coloring, or more than 10 grams of sugar per serving.

1 cup cereal
1 cup 2% milk, soy milk, Rice Dream, almond, or hemp milk
½ a banana or 4–5 strawberries, a handful of blueberries, or raisins, or cranberries
Handful of walnuts

Place the cereal in a bowl and top with the milk, your choice of fruit, and nuts.

***

Granola-Yogurt-Berry Parfait

Granola is a high-calorie cereal compared with other types. If you wish, you may use whole-grain cereals instead of the granola.

1 serving breakfast granola
½ cup good-quality yogurt, flavored if you like
½–1 cup seasonal berries
1 tablespoon sliced almonds
1 teaspoon honey (optional)

Place the cereal in the bottom of a bowl or cup, top with the yogurt, then berries, and finally the almonds. Drizzle honey on top if you like. Dip your spoon in all the way to the bottom and enjoy. You may replace the berries with any seasonal fruit.

***

Yogurt, a Handful of Nuts, and a Piece of Fruit

For those who don't want to go through the parfait-making process, just eat them all separately. You can skip the cereal here.

***

Packaged Instant Oatmeal

All you need is to follow the directions on the package. Mix a package of instant oatmeal with either milk or water, and either microwave or cook on the stove until set. Add some fresh or dried fruit, nuts (optional), a little more milk, and enjoy. This is the "fast food" of homemade breakfasts.

***

Zoom Hot Wheat Cereal

1 serving Zoom
¾ cup low-fat milk
Seasonal fruit, chopped
2 tablespoons sliced almonds or chopped walnuts (optional)
or
1 serving Zoom
¾ cup low-fat milk
1 tablespoon brown sugar or maple syrup
Seasonal fruit, chopped

Cook the cereal according to package directions in a bowl. Top with milk, and your choice of toppings.

***

Uncooked Rolled Oats

This is an excellent, nutritious breakfast that is great in hot weather.

½ cup old-fashioned rolled oats
1 cup milk, soy milk, or orange juice
1 tablespoon raisins
¼ apple, chopped
1 tablespoon almonds, preferably sliced or cut
Cinnamon (optional)

Combine and chill for 1 hour. Because the starch in the oats is uncooked, it tastes less sweet, so you can add a teaspoon of honey.

***

Eggs

This chapter includes a lot of egg recipes. Learning how to cook eggs will expand through your lifetime. Be sure to include a fruit or vegetable and whole-grain toast to round out this inexpensive and high protein meal. Served a variety of ways, eggs are full of protein and essential nutrients. Egg yolks tend to be high in cholesterol, though. One way to limit cholesterol is to mix one whole egg with one or two egg whites.

Remember about salmonella—wash your hands after touching raw eggs, and make sure the eggs are fully cooked, particularly if there is any news on salmonella.

***

Hard-Boiled Eggs

Place eggs in a saucepan and add water to cover the eggs by a couple of inches. Bring the water in the saucepan to a simmer and cook for 7 minutes. Remove the pan from the heat and allow them to cool for about 5 minutes. Peel and eat.

Hard-boiled eggs will keep in the refrigerator for about a week, as long as they have not been sitting out of the refrigerator for more than 2 hours. Hard boil 5-6 eggs at a time. This is a handy way to have a snack or quick meal available when you are hungry. Eggs can be eaten for breakfast or for lunch in a sandwich.

Note: One way to tell if an egg is hard boiled vs. raw is to "spin" the egg. On a countertop, a hard-boiled egg will spin rapidly. A raw egg is wobbly and doesn't spin well at all. This is a low-calorie, high-protein food.

***

Scrambled Eggs

1 teaspoon of canola oil or butter
2 eggs
Salt and pepper

In a small skillet, heat canola oil or butter. Crack open the eggs and add them to the pan. Using your wooden spoon, stir the eggs until the yolks and whites are mixed. Cook the eggs over medium to medium-low heat until they are just set. Season to taste with salt and pepper.

Serve with a slice of toast, a piece of fruit, and coffee or tea.

***

Poached Eggs

Bring a skillet of water to a slow simmer. Carefully crack eggs and slide them into the water. Don't worry if your egg spreads out in the water. Let the egg simmer in the water for 3–4 minutes or until the yolk is cooked the way you like it. Using a spoon or utensil that has slits in it to drain water, scoop the egg out of the water and serve.

***

Poached Egg on Toast

Toast a slice of your favorite whole-grain bread. Poach an egg until the whites are cooked but the yolk is still slightly runny. Place the egg on the toast and serve.

***

Sunny-Side-Up Eggs

This merely refers to cooking eggs in a skillet without turning them over. Place a small amount of oil in a skillet and warm over medium-low heat. Add eggs and place a lid on the skillet for about a minute or two. Remove the lid and check to see if the yolks are cooked the way you like them. If need be, let cook a little longer. Scoop them up with a spatula and plate them for eating.

***

Omelet

A basic omelet is an outside layer of whipped eggs folded over a filling inside. The filling may include vegetables, cheese, meats, seafood, or a combination.

A tablespoon of canola oil
2 whole eggs, or 1 whole egg and 2 egg whites
Salt and pepper
Dash of milk or water
Filling: see below

In a small nonstick skillet, heat the oil over medium heat. While the oil is heating, crack the eggs into a bowl and add salt, pepper, and dash of liquid. Whisk together until well blended. Add the eggs to the heated pan and swirl to coat the bottom of the pan with the egg.

As the eggs cook, lift the edges up so that the uncooked portion of the egg on top can run under and cook. When the egg is almost cooked through, add the filling and fold half of the eggs over on top of the filling. Turn the heat to low and place a lid over the skillet. Let the eggs and filling heat through for about a minute.

Serve omelet with fruit and a piece of toast or a serving of potatoes.

Omelet filling suggestions: Cook the filling in the oil prior to adding the whisked eggs. Once you turn it over and the top starts to harden, you can add some of your favorite cheese, which will melt.

- Vegetarian/Vegetable: ¼ cup chopped onions, peppers, and mushrooms, mixed.
- Vegetarian/Vegetable: 10 spears asparagus and 1 tablespoon parsley.
- Wild Mushrooms: ¼ cup mixed mushrooms that have been sautéed in a teaspoon of olive oil, shallots, salt, and pepper. A suggested mix includes 1 shitake mushroom, 2 brown and 2 white cremini mushrooms, chopped, and 1 teaspoon chopped shallot. Sauté all together until the mushrooms are soft, then add them to the omelet.
- Mexican: ½ Roma tomato, chopped; 1 tablespoon chopped onion; 1 tablespoon chopped cilantro; ½ minced jalapeno pepper; ½ ounce shredded jack cheese.
- Seafood: 4–5 cleaned and cooked shrimp, onions, cilantro.

***

Gashouse Egg

This is an old recipe offered to us by one of the editors of this book.

1 slice of whole wheat bread
1 egg
1 teaspoon of butter
Salt and pepper to taste

Butter the bread on both sides and with a small knife cut out a circular piece about 1 ½ " diameter. Heat a dry skillet and put the bread in it to fry. Immediately crack an egg into the hole in the bread, When the egg is beginning to firm up, flip the bread with the egg over and finish cooking it to create a combined egg-over-easy and toast.

***

Tomatoes with Scrambled Eggs

This recipe is great when you have an overripe tomato that can't be eaten fresh anymore.

1 teaspoon canola oil or butter
1 large tomato
2 eggs
Salt and pepper
White or whole-wheat pita bread

In a small skillet, heat canola oil or butter. Peel the tomato and slice it thinly. Cook on low-medium for 5 minutes until tomato turns into a soft paste. Crack the eggs and add them to the tomato. Using wooden spoon, stir the eggs until the eggs and the tomatoes are well mixed. Cook the eggs over medium to medium-low heat for about 2–3 minutes. Season to taste with salt and pepper. Cut the bread into two pockets and stuff it with eggs.

***

Scrambled Egg Wrap with Cherry Tomatoes

1 tablespoon shredded mozzarella cheese
1 sheet lavash or one wheat tortilla
2 eggs
1 teaspoon canola oil or butter
Handful cherry tomatoes, cut in half

1 teaspoon cilantro, chopped
Salt and pepper

Sprinkle the mozzarella on the lavash or tortilla and toast it 1 minute for lavash or 3 minutes for tortilla. Scramble the eggs in the canola oil or butter, add the cut cherry tomatoes and cilantro, then season with salt and pepper. Spread the mixture on the flat warm bread and roll it like in an aram sandwich or breakfast burrito. Cut 2½-inch slices and arrange on the plate.

***

Scrambled Tofu (Vegan)

You can use any vegetables! Green beans, peppers, eggplant, carrots, or whatever you like.

½ small onion
4–6 mushrooms
1–2 teaspoons olive oil
½ block (8 ounces) firm tofu
¼ teaspoon turmeric or paprika
Salt and pepper

Sauté the onions and mushrooms in a little bit of olive oil. Slice up the tofu and throw into the onions after they're done. Mash the tofu with a fork, and that'll give you the consistency of scrambled eggs. Dust it with turmeric or paprika, and that will give you the color of scrambled eggs and some flavor. Add some salt and pepper, and it will now taste like scrambled eggs. Serve with a bit of hot sauce and whole wheat toast, and you've got the entire scrambled egg experience. Tofu is 25% protein, compared with 12% for eggs.

***

Breakfast Burrito

This is easy to make once you've made any of the previous egg recipes. You can place scrambled eggs on top of a tortilla, sprinkle with cheese (or not), sprinkle with hot sauce (or not), fold the bottom, and bring in the sides. You can use aluminum foil to help maintain the shape; just don't bite any of the foil.

Here is a recipe for a *de-novo* breakfast burrito:

½ chopped red bell pepper, or beans, mushrooms, asparagus, spinach
½ medium onion, chopped
2 teaspoons olive oil
2 eggs
Salt and pepper
1 whole wheat, white, or corn tortilla

Sauté the vegetables in the olive oil until tender. Beat the eggs, add salt and pepper, and add to the vegetables. Cook the mixture until eggs are set, then place on the tortilla and fold.

***

French Toast

This is a great recipe if you have stale bread that is hard to eat. You turn it into a fluffy and tasty dish.

2 eggs
½ cup milk
Pinch of salt
3-4 slices of any bread, whole-wheat preferably
2 teaspoons oil or butter
Toppings:1 tablespoon maple syrup or jam, grated cheese, or sugar with cinnamon

Break the eggs into a wide, shallow bowl and mix with milk and salt. Place the slices of bread into the egg mix and let them soak on both sides (do not oversoak or the bread will crumble into the mixture). Heat a nonstick skillet and coat it with the ½ the oil (use more as needed for other slices). Once the skillet is hot, transfer the bread onto the skillet and cook until golden on the bottom. Then turn and cook the other side. When both sides are brown, place on a plate and serve hot with one of the toppings.

***

Potato Latkes

Surprise your Jewish friends with this traditional Jewish meal.

2 cups chopped potatoes
1 onion, chopped
2 eggs, beaten
1 teaspoon salt, dash of pepper, shake of cumin (optional)
2 tablespoons all-purpose flour
½ cup canola oil

Place potatoes and onion into a Cuisinart and mix until it looks like it is almost grated. Add the eggs, salt, pepper, and flour. Mix into a crude mass. Heat the oil in a large-bottom skillet until hot. Place large spoonfuls of potato mixture in the skillet, forming ½-inch-thick patties. Brown the patties on both sides, then remove from skillet and place on a paper towel to absorb the excess oil. Serve hot with applesauce.

***

Zucchini Patties

If your neighbor grows zucchini and brought you some, this is an easy way to use it.

2 cups shredded zucchini
1 clove garlic, finely chopped

2 eggs, beaten
1 teaspoon salt, dash of pepper, shake of cumin, and a dash of red pepper (optional)
3 tablespoons all-purpose flour
½ cup canola oil

Place the shredded zucchini (a Cuisinart will do the job) and garlic in a bowl. Add the eggs, seasonings, and flour. Mix into a crude mass. Heat the oil in a large-bottom skillet until hot. Place large spoonfuls of the mixture into it, pressing down with a fork and forming into ½-inch-thick patties. Cook until golden on one side and then turn them over, cooking until golden on the other. Remove from the pan and place on paper towels to absorb excess oil before serving.

***

Pancakes and Crepes

Pancakes and crepes are quite similar in their ingredients but different in thickness and presentation. When cooking, allow yourself to have a couple of bad ones until you get the hang of cooking them. Crepes are thinner and usually have more eggs, while pancakes have baking powder to make them fluffy.

Here is how to make pancakes from scratch:

1 cup all-purpose flour
1 teaspoon baking powder
1 teaspoon sugar
Pinch of salt
1 egg
1 cup milk
1 tablespoon butter or canola oil
Cooking spray or another tablespoon of oil

Combine dry ingredients in one bowl. Whisk the egg, milk, and the oil in another bowl, and then mix the parts (dry and wet ingredients) together. Spray a large skillet with cooking spray, or add the additional oil. Once it heats, add ¼-cup scoop of batter in plops into the skillet. Once bubbles appear on the surface of the pancakes and the edges look dry, it is time to flip them and cook the other side. Eat the pancakes warm with real maple syrup.

Crepes from Scratch

2 cups all-purpose flour
4 eggs
2 cups low-fat milk
½ teaspoon salt
3–4 tablespoons butter or oil

Mix all the ingredients in a blender. If the batter is too thick, add 1–2 tablespoons of water. Let the batter sit for 1 hour or even overnight. Refrigerating the batter is a good idea. To cook, pour ¼ cup into a large nonstick greased skillet and tilt it around to spread it evenly in the pan. Loosen the edges and flip it over. The other side cooks in about 20 seconds or less. Remove the thin crepe and set aside on a plate to cool. You can spread it with jam, hazelnut spread, melted chocolate, sliced bananas, or even leftovers from the night before, folding it like a homemade tortilla. In Russian culture, it is popular to fill crepes with cottage cheese and sugar. You can make them fancy by adding some red caviar and either rolling the crepe or folding it.

***

Peanut Butter Toast

If you are allergic to peanuts but like nut butters, you are in luck. These days most supermarkets carry a variety of nut butters, such as almond or cashew. However, a tablespoon of nut butter may contain around 200 calories. Use half that amount. Simply toast your favorite whole-grain bread and spread ½ tablespoon of peanut or other nut butter over while the toast is still hot.

***

Bagels and Cream Cheese

When you're buying bagels, you need to know that most bagels have 50–75 grams of simple carbs, and with cream cheese they provide more than 350 calories. There are a variety of sizes and nutritional quality, and frequently you will get too many calories from carbohydrates. However, here is an important concept: no one has ever gained weight from eating one bagel with cream cheese.

If you choose a whole-wheat bagel and low-fat cream cheese, then calories drop by 70–100 and the protein and fiber increase, maybe even double.

***

Muffins and Doughnuts

Everyone knows that these foods are high-calorie and low-nutrition foods. Most of the time, these foods provide little or no protein, fiber, or essential nutrients. Unless you can come up with a perfect recipe that is lower in calories, loaded with nutrition, contains a high amount of fiber, and is easy to prepare, consume these foods rarely. There are varieties of whole-grain muffin mixes on the market. You can make a dozen and have those in the mornings with a thin layer of butter.

Protein Smoothie

Your own smoothie might taste different than Jamba Juice but will be quite nutritious and filling. It will also be full of protein and antioxidants, and easy to make. Here is where you make use of your blender.

1 cup soy milk, almond milk, hemp milk, or regular low-fat milk
2 tablespoons ground flax (optional)
1 scoop protein powder
1 banana
Your choice of a pear, a peeled orange, an apple, or ½ cup berries

Blend all ingredients until smooth. Depending on the protein powder you use, it may impart a chalky feel to the smoothie. Also, flax adds a little crunch or grainy texture. No worries. This is filling and will hold you over for hours.

***

Fruit Smoothies

There is nothing as refreshing and simple as a fruit smoothie. Just put all of your fruits into a blender and mix. Experiment with a variety of fruits and find a combo that you like. If a smoothie is a little stiff, simply add some liquid, such as bubbly or still water, milk, juice, or crushed ice. If you are craving a fruit that is out of season, look in the freezer section of your grocery store. You will be amazed at the variety of fruits available for your smoothies.

To improve texture, you can add yogurt and/or banana to any of the recipes. To increase the satiety, add 1 tablespoon of protein powder or wheat germ. Here are some seasonal suggestions for smoothies.

Summer:

- 1 peach or nectarine, ½ cup plums, vanilla yogurt, and ½ cup ice, blended
- ½ cup raspberries or any other berries, yogurt, banana, 1 tablespoon protein powder or wheat germ, and ½ cup nonfat milk or soy milk

Autumn:

- 2 peaches, ½ cup pineapple, ½ cup yogurt, and ½ cup crushed ice, blended
- 1 apple, 1 kiwi, ½ cup vanilla yogurt, and ½ cup rice milk

Winter:

- ½ grapefruit, peeled and sectioned, 2 small tangerines, 1 banana, ½ cup orange juice, and 1 tablespoon wheat germ, blended
- ½ papaya, ½ banana, ¼ cup mineral water, ½ cup vanilla yogurt, blended.

Spring:

- ½ cup pineapple, 1 mango, cut into chunks (frozen is great), ½ cup yogurt, and ½ cup ice, blended.
- your choice of mixed frozen berries, about 1 cup, ½ cup low-fat yogurt, 1–2 teaspoons honey, 1 tablespoon protein powder, blended

***

2. Sandwiches

"Too few people understand a really good sandwich."

James Beard

"I don't need music, lobster or wine

Whenever your eyes look into mine;

The things I long for are simple and few:

A cup of coffee, a **sandwich***—and you!"*

Billy Rose

Some sort of a sandwich is known in every culture, and everyone loves them. They are easy to prepare and can be eaten for breakfast, lunch, or dinner. When you make a good sandwich—that is, one that you like and that is nutritionally sound—it will fill you up for hours.

Every sandwich consists of a top and bottom layer of bread, preferably whole grain. Choosing your bread is very important. There are varieties of whole-grain, multigrain, rice flour, potato flour, gluten-free, and also many white breads that have no nutritional value. Look for the fiber and the protein content. The higher the fiber and protein content, the higher the bread quality. The longer the ingredient list, the lower the quality is for the bread you're looking at.

What goes in between the bread slices is a personal choice of proteins, condiments, and vegetables. Proteins can be any meat, fish, poultry, nut butter, cheese, hummus, or tofu. Condiments may include ketchup, avocado, mustard, mayo, pesto, hummus, vegetable spread, pepper spread, or a vinaigrette dressing. Vegetables may be lettuce, tomato, sprouts, avocado, grilled peppers, pea shoots, onions, arugula, zucchini, portabella mushrooms, eggplant, etc. A sandwich can easily become a staple just like the hamburger, which is a modified sandwich. Your favorite foods in a sandwich determine for you whether you will eat it regularly.

Note: When using mayonnaise, don't smother the bread. Though more and more mayos on the market are free of bad ingredients, use them sparingly.

For a complete meal, plan on serving your sandwich with a piece of fruit or a salad, milk, tea, coffee, or water. You can also have a small chocolate chip or oatmeal cookie if you still feel hungry.

***

Turkey Sandwich with Swiss Cheese

2 slices whole-grain bread, toasted optional
Mustard and/or mayo
2 ounces thinly sliced cooked turkey meat
1-ounce slice Swiss cheese
2 slices tomato
1 large lettuce leaf, romaine or iceberg
Alfafa sprouts (optional)
Red onion, thinly sliced (optional)

Spread the bread with a small amount of mustard and/or mayo. Layer bread with the turkey meat, cheese slice, tomato, and lettuce, and top with the second slice of bread. Add optional ingredients if desired.

***

Tuna Salad Sandwich (serves 2)

1 can water-packed tuna, drained (each 5-ounce can is 2 servings)
2 tablespoons light mayonnaise
½ celery stick, strings removed and chopped finely
Salt and pepper
4 slices whole-grain bread, toasted
4 lettuce leaves
2 or 4 slices tomato

Drain the water from the tuna in the can and place the drained tuna in a bowl. With a fork, break down the chunks of tuna and mix with the mayonnaise and celery. Season to taste with salt and pepper.

On a slice of toasted bread, layer a lettuce leaf, half of the tuna salad, 1 or 2 slices of tomato, and another lettuce leaf. Top with the second slice of bread.

***

Roast Chicken Sandwich (serves 2)

A half chicken breast, cooked, sliced
4 slices toasted whole-grain bread
2 tablespoons pesto
2 (1-ounce) slices provolone cheese
Tomato slices
Lettuce leaves

Thinly slice the half chicken breast and divide it into two servings. For each sandwich, spread the toasted bread with 1 tablespoon pesto. Layer the chicken slices, cheese, tomato and lettuce. Top with the other bread slice.

***

Fried Egg Sandwich

Mustard
2 slices whole-grain bread, toasted
1 egg "fried" in a nonstick skillet with no oil
Tomato slices
Lettuce
Salt and pepper

Spread mustard on your toasted bread. Layer the egg, tomato, and lettuce, and season with salt and pepper. Top with second toast slice. This same sandwich can be made with a hard-boiled sliced egg.

***

Mediterranean Pita Sandwich

Pita, or pocket bread, these days is available in almost every store and is a great way of creating a sandwich.

1 large pita bread, sliced in half to create two pockets
3 tablespoons hummus, plain or flavored
Lettuce leaves
Tomato
Cucumber
Alfalfa sprouts
Slice of Havarti or other cheese (optional)
2 ounces thinly sliced lunch meat (optional)

In each half pocket, spread hummus to moisten the bread. Add the rest of the ingredients into each pocket and enjoy.

Other suggested fillings for pita sandwiches:
* 3 ounces roast chicken, chopped (use leftovers if you have them), sliced cucumber, red pepper, lettuce, tomato, and mustard

- 3 tablespoons tzatziki (a cucumber, garlic, herb, and yogurt blend), sliced red pepper, lettuce, alfalfa sprouts, and turkey lunch meat if desired
- 2 ounces thinly sliced teriyaki chicken or roast beef, lettuce, chopped scallions, and a sprinkling of sesame seeds on top
- Meatballs (see the recipe in the pasta section), lettuce, green peppers
- Sardines, hard-boiled egg, red onions
- Smoked salmon, cream cheese, arugula, and asparagus
- Refried black beans, sour cream, thinly shredded cheese

***

Peanut Butter, Banana, and Honey Sandwich

2 slices whole-grain toast
1 tablespoon peanut butter (almond butter or other nut butter is good, too)
½ banana, thinly sliced
Honey

On 1 slice of the toasted bread, spread the nut butter. Layer on top the banana slices and drizzle with honey. Top with the second slice of bread.

***

Peanut Butter and Jelly Sandwich

2 slices whole-grain bread
1 tablespoon peanut butter (or other nut butter)
1 tablespoon jam

On one slice of bread, spread the nut butter. On top of that, spread the jam. Top with second slice of bread. That is it!

***

Grilled Cheese Sandwich

Warm sandwiches are great in winter and can be eaten as a part of a dinner. The grilled cheese sandwich is the basic version of more fancy warm sandwiches.

3 slices cheese
2 slices bread
1 teaspoon butter

Place the cheese slices between two slices of any bread and spread the butter on of the outside of the bread slices. Fry them on a nonstick skillet. The bread becomes crisp and the cheese melts. This is the simplest of all sandwiches and is loved universally. Pair it with a bowl of organic tomato or roasted pepper soup (premade from a can or a carton) and a piece of fruit, and you have a tasty, extremely inexpensive, yummy dinner. A dinner like this at home will cost you under $3. No wonder cheese sandwiches were very popular during World War II.

***

Panini

An Italian sandwich commonly made with ciabbata or rosetta breads.

½ loaf Italian bread

Stuff the bread with your choice of sliced mozzarella, prosciutto, peppers, basil, tomatoes, spinach, portabella mushroom, figs, and whatever tastes good to you. Brush both sides of the bread with olive oil and grill on a nonstick pan on both sides. You can Americanize the panini and put eggs and bacon between two slices of sourdough bread.

***

Tortillas and Roll-Ups

Whenever you have leftover meat (chicken, beef, ground meats), all you need to do is add side condiments to make a full meal with a "make-your-own burrito." Please don't feel intimidated by the list of condiments. Pick and choose what you like! This is a hit with almost everyone I know. See what you think.

Whole grain tortillas
Leftover chicken (shredded), sliced beef, ground turkey, or ground beef; or skip the meat and make this a non-animal burrito!
Chopped cilantro
Chopped red onion
Chopped tomato
Finely grated cheddar or jack cheese
Chopped avocado or guacamole
Fresh-cut salsa or store-bought red salsa, green or tomatillo salsa, mango salsa, etc.
Plain low-fat yogurt or sour cream
Roasted vegetables, such as red peppers, onions, sweet potato or butternut squash, and zucchini
Black or pinto beans (these can be whole, mashed, or refried)
Finely shredded cabbage or lettuce

Place a tortilla on your plate and spread with some of the beans. Layer the meat if using, and add any of the rest of the toppings that you like. Roll the tortillas up and around the fillings.

Popular combinations include:

Turkey Burrito: Tortilla; ¼ cup nonfat refried beans; topped with ¼ cup finely shredded lettuce; ¼ cup cooked ground turkey seasoned with Mexican spices (see recipe below); ¼ avocado, chopped; chopped tomato; 2 tablespoons shredded jack cheese; and fresh salsa.

Beef Burrito: Tortilla; ¼ cup mashed black beans; 2–3 ounces thinly sliced grilled flank steak or other leftover steak; ¼ cup finely shredded cabbage; cilantro; 2 tablespoons guacamole; chopped tomato; 2 tablespoons shredded sharp cheddar; and a dollop of light sour cream or plain yogurt.

Vegetarian Burrito: Tortilla; ¼ cup black beans; ¼ cup roasted butternut squash and onions; shredded lettuce; 2 tablespoons shredded jack cheese or 2 tablespoons light sour cream.

Note: Notice how we haven't mentioned putting rice in the burrito? White rice acts as a filler for the burritos and doesn't add much nutrition. In fact, you get all the starch you need with the tortilla, so you don't need the rice unless you are very hungry.

Mexican Seasoned Ground Turkey Meat

This seasoned turkey meat is great in burritos and tacos, or stir some into scrambled eggs with shredded cheddar on top for breakfast. Because it uses an entire package of ground turkey, plan on using this over several days.

1 package lean ground turkey, 1¼ pounds
½ teaspoon each ground cumin, dried oregano, dried thyme, garlic powder, salt, and pepper
2 teaspoons ground chili powder

In a skillet, heat a small amount of canola or olive oil and add the ground turkey. Season the meat and cook until it is no longer pink. Break up the turkey meat into small pieces and stir occasionally while cooking. This makes 4–6 servings.

***

Chicken Quesadilla

1 ounce cheddar or jack cheese, shredded
2 ounces shredded chicken (leftovers work well here)
1 whole-grain flour tortilla
Salsa, your favorite kind

Sprinkle the cheese and chicken over half of the tortilla and fold the other half over. Cook the tortilla in a dry skillet over medium heat until the cheese is melted. Serve with salsa.

***

Cheese Quesadilla

2 tortillas, whole grain preferably
Mixed shredded Mexican cheese
A pat of butter or vegetable spread

Cover one tortilla with cheese generously and top it with the other tortilla. Lightly spread the butter or the vegetable spread on the top tortilla and place the quesadilla into a toaster oven or broiler for 3–5 minutes until the top tortilla is golden brown and cheese is melted. Let it cool and cut into 4 parts. Enjoy with salad or soup. This may also be cooked in a nonstick pan for 3–5 minutes on each side.

***

Cheese and Vegetable Quesadilla

½ cup each sliced onion and peppers
1 ounce cheddar or jack cheese, shredded
1 whole-grain tortilla
Salsa, your favorite kind

Spray a small skillet with Pam cooking spray and cook the onions and peppers over medium heat until softened and fragrant. Place the cooked vegetables and shredded cheese on one half of the tortilla and fold the other half over. Cook in a dry skillet until the cheese is melted. Serve with salsa.

***

Lavash (Flat Bread) Roll-up—Aram Sandwiches

The correct name for the bread is "lavash," not "lavosh" or "la-wash" or any other weird name. Lavash is traditional Armenian bread, made of flour, water, and salt. While the Armenian lavash is very thin, in the United States lavash is thicker and more suitable for aram sandwiches. Making an aram sandwich is easy and quick, and you can change the ingredients according to whatever you have handy. Just master the technique and then use your creativity.

1 sheet white or preferably whole-wheat or whole-grain lavash
2 tablespoons light cream cheese
3 ounces thinly sliced lunch meat
Lettuce or spinach
Cheese slices (optional)
Thinly sliced red onion (optional)

Spread the lavash bread with cream cheese. Layer the lunch meat, follow with lettuce, then cheese, then onion, leaving about 1 inch on 1 end with just cream cheese. Roll up the bread and fillings, starting at the opposite end from the plain cream cheese edge. Keep it rolled for 15 minutes in plastic wrap, and then slice the roll-up and serve. You may keep it overnight in the refrigerator. Cut it into 2½-inch slices.

Other suggested combinations for lavash roll-ups:
- Salmon-flavored light cream cheese, thinly sliced red onion, capers, and a hard-boiled egg white, chopped
- Vegetable-flavored light cream cheese, shredded carrots, peppers, thinly sliced onion, alfalfa sprouts, tomato, and lettuce

- Goat cheese and a mix of roasted vegetables (for example, squash, eggplant, peppers, and onions)
- Hummus with roasted vegetables, spinach, and green onions.
- Peanut butter, jelly, and some crunchy cereal
- Honey, butter, and bananas or any other fruit

* * *

3. Salads

Today, salads encompass a wide variety of dishes; green salads, potato salads, legumes and meats, pasta salads, etc. Use your imagination! Salads can range from being a light side dish to a calorie-dense main course.

There are some general rules. If your salad is a side dish, then you need a foundation—greens (lettuce, mixed greens, or spinach), other veggies, croutons, etc.—and a salad dressing. If the salad is meant to be a main course, then you need to add protein, such as chicken, ham, turkey, fish, tofu, or beans. You can also add starches like potatoes, rice, couscous, or quinoa. If you don't want the hassle of making dressing, use store bought.

William Shakespeare called his younger years his "salad days." Enjoy your salads while living your salad days!

***

Green House Salad (per person)

1 cup or more of washed and torn lettuce (this can be a mixture of baby lettuces, spring mix, romaine, butter lettuce, green and/or red leaf lettuce)
A few cucumber slices
A small tomato, cut into wedges
Salad dressing (see Salad Dressings section)

Place all ingredients in a bowl and toss with 1 tablespoon of basic vinaigrette, balsamic vinaigrette, or any other dressing of your choice.

A green salad should be part of most dinners. You can fancy the basic salad with a variety of your favorite vegetables and fruits. A tablespoon of chopped nuts can be added. Pepper slices, sliced scallions, mushrooms, broccoli florets, arugula, endive, mandarin orange slices, dried cranberries, avocado, strawberries (fresh or dry), pears, apples, etc., can all be successfully used in a lot of different combinations. ½ ounce of Feta, blue cheese and Asiago cheeses will add to the flavor and make it richer.

Note: Nuts and cheeses are high in fat and calories. If you wish to keep your calorie count down, it is best to limit these choices. Avocados and nuts are high in fat, but rich in good and healthful oils. ¼ of an avocado or 2 tablespoons nuts would be a maximum serving..

***

Basic Vinaigrette

Salad dressings are composed of an oil, an acid, and seasoning. For the oils, the best to use is extra virgin olive oil or canola oil. The acids can be vinegar or citrus juice. Different vinegars have varied flavors. White wine vinegars, red wine vinegars, and rice wine vinegars are all available in most markets. The seasonings we use are the basic salt and pepper. You can add other herbs and spices such as thyme, powdered or Dijon mustard, or garlic to vary the taste, but that is up to you. One thing about salad dressings, you can always vary the ratios of ingredients to make a dressing that you like. For example, you can use 3 parts oil to 1 part vinegar for a less tart dressing. The following is a 2 parts oil to 1 part vinegar dressing. You don't need to add too much dressing on a salad. Toss your lettuces well so that each leaf has just a hint of flavor from the dressing.

¼ cup olive oil or canola oil
2 tablespoons vinegar (white wine vinegar, red wine vinegar, rice wine vinegar, etc.)

1 teaspoon lemon juice
Salt and pepper
1 teaspoon Dijon mustard (optional)
1 clove garlic, mashed (optional)

Whisk all together in a small bowl. Or, even easier, put all ingredients in a jar with a lid. Shake vigorously to mix. Toss with your salad of choice. If you would like, you can also add a pinch of sugar or honey to sweeten or soften the dressing.

***

Balsamic Vinaigrette

¾ cup olive oil
¼ cup balsamic vinegar
1 tablespoon chopped garlic (optional)
 ½ teaspoon salt
½ teaspoon freshly ground black pepper
1 teaspoon brown sugar (optional)
Blue cheese or feta cheese (optional added to salad)

Place all the ingredients except the cheese in a screw-top jar and shake to combine. Taste and adjust the seasonings. Top your salad with optional blue cheese, add a couple tablespoons of the dressing with your desired salad ingredients, and toss gently to coat all ingredients. Serve immediately. If not using dressing right away, cover and refrigerate, whisking or shaking again before use.

***

Caesar Salad (serves 4-6)

Head of romaine lettuce, leaves washed and dried
½ cup croutons
¼ cup finely grated Parmesan cheese

Caesar salad dressing (see below)
Lemon

Add the lettuce to a salad bowl along with the croutons and Parmesan cheese. Toss with enough salad dressing to moisten. Squeeze lemon juice over all. Toss again. You may add more grated Parmesan if you wish.

Caesar Salad Dressing (makes about ¾ cup)

½ cup olive oil
1-2 garlic cloves, minced
3 tablespoons white wine vinegar
Dash of Worcestershire sauce
Pinch of dry mustard
¼ cup finely grated Parmesan cheese
Salt and pepper
Squeeze of lemon (optional)

Place the olive oil and garlic in a jar with a lid. Let sit for about 15 minutes so that the garlic flavors the oil. Add the rest of the ingredients and shake vigorously to mix. Sample the dressing and adjust the seasonings. If you like a more lemony dressing, add lemon juice. If you like a stronger flavor, add more Worcestershire. If you don't have fresh garlic, use dried garlic powder.

***

Homemade Salad Bar (serves 2)

Just like you pile greens, vegetables, and meats in your bowl at a salad bar, do the same with your homemade salad. Check the refrigerator and pantry. Imagine a painting palette and you are the artist who needs to create an artwork. Make every salad a masterpiece. All of the ingredients in the following salad could be substituted for something similar.

½ cup cannelini beans, rinsed and drained (kidney or garbanzo beans)
1 cup diced cooked chicken breast (ham or turkey)
½ cup canned corn, rinsed and dried (green peas or slices of cooked potatoes)
1 cup cherry tomatoes
¼ cup crumbled feta cheese
1 cup lettuce (iceberg, butternut, arugula, or spinach)
½ cup radicchio leaves (optional)
2 tablespoons Basic Vinaigrette
½ cup chopped fresh basil and parsley

Combine beans, chicken, corn, tomatoes, and cheese in a bowl. Place the greens and radicchio leaves on a plate and put the chicken and bean mix on top of them. Sprinkle with dressing and garnish with basil and parsley. P.S. You don't need to add all of the ingredients and you can certainly experiment with others that you like!

***

Mexican Cabbage Slaw (serves 4 or more)

1 small green cabbage, very thinly sliced
1 small jicama root, peeled, cut into thin sticks
½ red or white onion, thinly sliced
A large handful of cilantro leaves, stems removed
Lime Vinaigrette (see below)
Salt and pepper to taste

Mix together the cabbage, jicama, onion, and cilantro in a salad bowl. Add ¼ cup of Lime Vinaigrette and toss all together. Season with salt and pepper. More dressing may be added if needed.

***

Lime Vinaigrette

1 garlic clove, minced
3 tablespoons canola oil
2 tablespoons lime juice
Salt and pepper to taste

In a small bowl, place garlic and oil together and let sit for a few minutes. Then add the lime juice, salt, and pepper. Whisk together well and toss with Mexican Cabbage Slaw.

***

Chinese Cabbage Salad (serves 6 or more)

1 head cabbage, finely shredded
1 bunch cilantro, stems removed
1 bunch green onions, sliced
1 cucumber, peeled, quartered lengthwise, and sliced thinly
Celery (optional)
Roasted sesame seeds or sliced almonds (optional)
1 package Nissan or Sapporo Ichiban noodles
Asian-Style Salad Dressing (see below)

In a large bowl add the finely shredded cabbage, cilantro leaves, green onions, cucumber, and celery and sesame seeds if using. Crumble the ramen noodles and add to the salad. Toss with salad dressing to your taste.

Asian-Style Salad Dressing (makes about ½ cup)

⅓ cup canola oil
3 tablespoons rice wine vinegar
1 teaspoon sesame oil
Salt and pepper
Honey

Whisk together all ingredients or shake them up in a jar. Taste to see if you need more honey, salt, or pepper.

***

Simple Seasoned Sliced Cucumbers

1 cucumber, peeled and sliced
Rice wine vinegar
Salt and pepper

In a bowl, sprinkle the cucumber slices with vinegar. Season to taste with salt and pepper. These quick "pickles" are a refreshing side dish for many meals.

***

Cucumber, Tomato, and Pineapple Salad with Asian Dressing (serves 3)

1 small garlic clove, minced
Pinch of salt
1 tablespoon fresh lime juice
1 teaspoon sugar
¼ teaspoon soy sauce
1 tablespoon canola oil
½ small jalapeno chile, minced, including seeds
½ seedless cucumber, halved lengthwise, then thinly sliced
1 cup pineapple, peeled, sliced ½-inch thick (cut into same size pieces as the cucumber)
¼ cup chopped fresh cilantro
2 tablespoons chopped fresh mint
1 medium tomato, cut into ½-inch wedges

Whisk together garlic, salt, lime juice, sugar, soy sauce, and oil until sugar and salt are dissolved. In a bowl, mix together the jalapeno chile, cucumber, pineapple, cilantro, and mint. Add the prepared vegetables to the dressing and toss to coat. Top with tomato wedges. Season to taste with a little more salt if needed.

***

Heirloom Tomato Salad with Olives and Basil (serves 4)

Lettuce greens
½ cup chopped red onion
¼ cup chopped fresh basil
16 thick slices of a variety of colorful heirloom tomatoes, halved
3 tablespoons balsamic vinegar
2 tablespoons water
1 tablespoon olive oil
2 tablespoon finely chopped Nicoise olives
1 garlic clove, crushed
¼ teaspoon sea salt
Pinch of black pepper

Place lettuce greens on a platter and sprinkle half of the onion and fresh basil over. Arrange the tomato slice halves over the lettuce and basil. Top with the remaining basil and onion. Mix together the balsamic vinegar, water, olive oil, chopped olives, garlic, salt, and pepper. Drizzle over the tomatoes and serve.

***

Mixed Summer Vegetable Salad

3–4 large ripe tomatoes
1 red or yellow bell pepper
1 green bell pepper
1 cucumber
Thinly sliced red onions (optional)

Fresh basil
Salt and pepper

Cut all the ingredients into the bowl, and add salt and pepper to taste. This salad doesn't require any oil or vinegar because the juice from the tomatoes and the added salt serve as dressing. Some great additions to this salad are a grilled cheese sandwich, pilaf with chicken, or beef kabobs.

***

Caprese Salad

3 vine-ripe tomatoes, ¼-inch-thick slices
1 pound fresh mozzarella, ¼-inch-thick slices
20–30 leaves (about 1 bunch) fresh basil
Extra virgin olive oil for drizzling
Coarse salt and pepper

Simply layer alternating slices of tomatoes and mozzarella, adding a basil leaf between each, on a large, shallow platter. Drizzle the salad with extra virgin olive oil and season with salt and pepper, to taste. For a variation on this theme, you may try sprinkling capers and small olives over all.

***

Black Bean Salad (2 or more servings)

1 15-ounce can black beans, drained and rinsed
½ red, yellow, or orange bell pepper, cut into ½-inch pieces
¼ cup diced red onion or 4 scallions, chopped
½ cup frozen corn, defrosted
¼ cup chopped cilantro
2 tablespoons Basic Vinaigrette or Lime Vinaigrette (see recipes above)

Toss all together in a bowl. This dish keeps for several days in the refrigerator. It pairs perfectly with grilled meats or as a luncheon side dish.

***

White Bean Salad with Roasted Tomatoes and Garlic (serves 6–8 as a side dish)

½ package dried white beans, such as navy
½ yellow onion, chopped
1 whole head garlic, top trimmed off to expose cloves
1 pound Roma tomatoes
1 pint mixed-color small cherry tomatoes
Olive oil
Salt (use coarse salt such as sea or kosher style), pepper, sugar
1 bunch fresh basil leaves

Place the beans in a large sauce pan and fill with water to about 1 inch over the beans. Bring to a boil on the stove top and let cook for 15 minutes. Turn the heat off the beans and allow them to cool completely. Drain the beans and place them back in the pan. Add fresh water to cover by 2 inches. Add the chopped onion and tuck the head of garlic into the beans. Bring to a boil, lower heat, and simmer until beans are just tender, about 1 or 1½ hours. More water may be added if it gets too low. If you overcook the beans, they will become mushy!

While the beans are cooking, slice the Roma tomatoes into quarters and place on a baking sheet with a rim. Add the small tomatoes and generously drizzle all with olive oil. Sprinkle several pinches of coarse salt, pepper, and sugar over and toss them to make sure the tomatoes are thoroughly coated and seasoned. Place them in an oven at 325 degrees for 45 minutes or until the tomatoes are softened and glazed. Remove from the oven and let cool.

When the beans have cooled, remove the garlic head and set it aside. Drain the beans and place in a bowl. Squeeze the garlic juice and pulp out of the head into the beans. Discard the used-up head of garlic. Add the roasted tomatoes to the beans and scrape any extra juices into them. Stir all together and test to see if the beans need more salt and pepper. Add ¼ cup chopped basil leaves (or more) into the beans and stir again. For decoration, place basil florettes on top of the beans to serve.

***

Lentil Salad with Tomatoes and Herbs (serves 4–6 as a side dish)

This lentil dish is very versatile in that it can accommodate more vegetables if you like (diced cucumbers and red peppers, for example) as well as different herbs, such as parsley and cilantro.

3 cups water
½ teaspoon salt
1 cup dried lentils, preferably the small French ones
1 large clove garlic, chopped
2 cups fresh tomatoes, diced
½ cup or more thinly sliced scallions
¼ cup chopped dill
¼ cup chopped basil
3 tablespoons cider or red wine vinegar
3 tablespoons olive oil
Salt and pepper to taste

Bring water and salt to boil. Add the lentils and garlic and boil until lentils are tender but not mushy, 15–25 minutes. Drain. In a bowl, add the rest of the ingredients to the hot lentils and season to taste. Enjoy!

***

Quinoa Salad with White Cheddar (serves 4–6)

1 cup quinoa, rinsed
2 ounces sharp white cheddar, cut into small cubes
¼ cup parsley
3 scallions, chopped
Light vinaigrette, or just olive oil
Salt and pepper

Cook the quinoa according to package directions. When done, drain the quinoa and add to a bowl. Mix in the cheese, parsley, and scallions, and toss with vinaigrette until just moistened. Season to taste with salt and pepper.

***

Tabbouleh

This is a Lebanese summer salad that is somewhat heavy on chopping but always turns out well. You probably would make it for a party and not for just a dinner salad.

1 cup bulgur
3 tomatoes, seeded and chopped
2 cucumbers, peeled and chopped
3 green onions, chopped
2 cloves garlic, minced
1 cup chopped fresh parsley
1 green bell pepper, chopped
⅓ cup fresh mint leaves
1½ teaspoons salt
½ cup lemon juice
½ cup olive oil

Place bulgur in bowl and cover with 2 cups boiling water. Soak for 30 minutes; drain and squeeze out excess water.

In a mixing bowl, combine bulgur, tomatoes, cucumbers, onions, garlic, parsley, bell pepper, mint, salt, lemon juice, and olive oil. Toss and refrigerate for at least 4 hours before serving. Toss again prior to serving. You may add another finely chopped tomato if you like.

***

Bulgur or Wheat Berry Salad with Tangerine (4 servings)

½ cup bulgur or wheat berries, cooked
½ cup diced red pepper
½ cup diced red onion
½ cup sliced almonds
½ cup chopped parsley
The juice of 2 tangerines
1 tablespoon olive oil
Salt and pepper to taste

Toss all together. Make in advance so the flavors meld.

***

Fruit Salads

Fruit salads can be made from any variety of fruits that are in season. Canned fruits are a good standby when you crave a piece of fruit that is currently out of season or transported from another part of the world. Check your local farmer's markets or grocers and buy local and fresh produce.

The following salads are just a few of the many combinations that you may come up with.

Contemporary Ambrosia Salad (serves 4)

2 oranges, peeled and chopped
2 cups pineapple, cut into same size pieces as the oranges

1 banana, sliced
2 tablespoons shredded dried coconut (optional)
A small splash of orange juice
¼ teaspoon almond extract
Almond slices

Combine all the fruit in a bowl and stir in the orange juice and almond extract. Serve with sliced almonds sprinkled over.

***

Mixed Fruit Salad (serves 4)

1 red apple, peeled, cored, and cut into 1-inch pieces
1 Asian pear, cut into cubes the same size as the apple
2–4 tangerines, peeled and sectioned
A handful of strawberries, cut in half
A sprinkling of sliced almonds

Mix all together and serve. No dressing is needed. If you plan on keeping this in the refrigerator for a few days, a squeeze of lemon or lime juice over the apples and pears keeps them from discoloring.

***

Honeydew Melon with Blackberries

This color combination looks beautiful on any table with the contrasting colors of the fruit. Even the most novice cook can take advantage of the fruits of any season to cash in on the wow factor of colorful fruit.

1 sweet green honeydew melon, peeled, seeded, and cut into cubes
2 pints fresh blackberries

Place the honeydew melon and 1 pint of blackberries in a serving bowl and gently mix with your hands. Sprinkle the second pint of blackberries over the top. You may decorate this with a sprig of mint for that extra touch.

***

Fall Fruit Salad (serves 4)

2 apples
3 pears
3 ounces candied pecans or plain roasted pecans
¼ cup dried cranberries
Orange juice
Salt and pepper to taste

Peel, core, and chop apples and pears into cubes. Place in a bowl and add the pecans, cranberries, and just enough orange juice to moisten the fruit. You may add salt and pepper if you desire.

***

4. Vegetable Side Dishes

The following are colorful and flavorful vegetable dishes that round out your meal. Vegetables can be steamed, sautéed, fried, baked, or grilled. The exact same vegetable will taste differently and will contain very different amount of calories depending on the way you cook it.

***

Asparagus (per serving)

5–7 stalks of asparagus

Fill a skillet halfway with water. Bring the water to a gentle simmer on the stove. While waiting for the water to heat, "snap" the tough ends of your asparagus stalks off and discard the ends. Add the trimmed asparagus to the hot water and cook until just tender, about 3–5 minutes. Remove from the water immediately and serve with salt and pepper.

***

Asparagus Salad (serves 4)

1 bunch asparagus, tough ends snapped off
Balsamic Vinaigrette, see recipe above

¼ cup diced red pepper
¼ cup walnuts or pecans, chopped

Bring a skillet of water to simmer and cook the asparagus until just tender, about 3–5 minutes. Remove from the water and place on a serving platter.

Mix together ½ cup of balsamic vinaigrette with the red pepper and nuts. Drizzle over the asparagus and serve. This recipe can be made several hours before serving. Just keep refrigerated until you are ready.

***

Steamed Broccoli (per serving)

Large handful of broccoli florets
Lemon, salt, and pepper

Place a steamer basket in a saucepan and add about 1 or 2 inches of water to the pan. Bring the water to a simmer and add the broccoli florets to the steamer basket. Place a lid on the pan and cook for about 3 minutes or until the broccoli is tender. Serve with a squeeze of lemon and salt and pepper to taste.

***

Steamed Brussels Sprouts (per serving)

5–7 brussels sprouts
Butter (optional), salt, and pepper

Trim off the stem end of the Brussels sprouts and pull off any discolored leaves. Place a steamer basket into a saucepan with a lid. Add 1–2 inches of water to the pan and bring to a boil. Add the sprouts to the steamer basket and cover with the lid. Steam for 7–9 minutes or until the sprouts are tender.

Toss the Brussels sprouts with a teaspoon of butter and salt and pepper to taste.

***

Sautéed Brussels Sprouts (serves 2)

1 tablespoon olive oil
10-12 brussels sprouts, trimmed and sliced very thin
2 tablespoons finely chopped walnuts
Salt, pepper, and lemon

Heat about a tablespoon of olive oil in a skillet and add the thinly sliced Brussels sprouts and walnuts. Stir while cooking. When the sprouts are tender, about 3 minutes, remove from heat and season to taste with salt, pepper, and a squeeze of lemon if desired.

***

Steamed Green Beans (per serving)

10–12 green beans, ends trimmed off
Salt and pepper

Add an inch or two of water to a saucepan with a steamer basket and a lid. Heat the water to a simmer and add the green beans to the steamer basket. Cover and cook for about 3–5 minutes or until the green beans are tender. Season to taste with salt and pepper,
For an extra flavor boost, steamed green beans are delicious with lemon butter. Melt a tablespoon of butter and add a couple drops of fresh lemon juice to it. Stir together and mix into the green beans.

***

Steamed Cauliflower (serves 4-6)

1 head cauliflower, cut or broken into even-sized florets
Salt and pepper
Butter (optional)

Place a steamer basket in a saucepan and add about 1 inch of water. Bring the water to a boil and add the cauliflower florets. Place a lid on the pan and cook for 5 minutes or until the cauliflower is tender. (A knife or fork poked into the vegetable will easily cut the vegetable, but make sure you don't overcook it to the falling-apart state).

Drain the water from the cauliflower and season to taste with salt and pepper. You may add a tablespoon or so of butter if you wish.

***

Corn on the Cob (per serving)

One ear of corn, outer leaves and strings removed

Bring a large pot of water to a boil and add the ear of corn. Let it cook for just a couple of minutes and remove it from the water. Bite in and enjoy!

***

Carrot Coins with Butter and Brown Sugar (per serving)

1 large carrot, scrubbed and cut into coins
1 teaspoon brown sugar
1 teaspoon butter

In a saucepan, cook the carrots in water until just tender. Drain the water from the carrots and stir in the brown sugar and butter.

***

Sauteed Leeks (per serving)

1 leek, discolored outer leaves pulled off, ends trimmed
1 tablespoon olive oil
1 tablespoon butter
Salt and pepper

Slice the leek into ¼-inch rounds. Make sure to clean out any noticeable dirt in the leeks.

Heat olive oil and butter in a skillet over low heat. Add the leeks and cook slowly until they are quite soft, about 15 minutes. Season with salt and pepper.

Sauteed leeks can be served over meats, added into mashed potatoes or into egg dishes, or served as a simple side dish.

***

Sautéed Mushrooms (per serving)

Sautéed mushrooms can be served over meats or as a simple side dish.

1 tablespoon olive oil
1 tablespoon butter
1 shallot, minced
1 small garlic clove, minced
¼ pound mushrooms, cleaned, stems trimmed and discarded, and sliced
2 tablespoons red wine
Salt and pepper

Melt the oil and butter together in a skillet and sauté the shallot and garlic for about 30 seconds. Add the mushrooms and cook over low heat until they are soft. Add the red wine and cook for a few minutes longer. Season to taste with salt and pepper.

***

Potatoes and Mushrooms

2 large potatoes, sliced thinly
2 tablespoons olive oil
1 onion, sliced
1 cup white or cremini mushrooms, cleaned, stems trimmed and discarded, and sliced
1 small garlic clove, minced
Salt and pepper

Cook the potatoes for 5 minutes in a small amount of hot water. If there is any liquid left, drain it off.   Add the olive oil and cook for another 5 minutes, then add the onions, mushrooms, and garlic. Mix and cook for another 8–10 minutes.

***

Chard, Collards, and Kale

These are all dark, large-leafed greens which have a strong, earthy flavor and are power foods for your body. The leaves need to be rinsed of any sand before cooking. These are great in stir-fries, sautéed in olive oil and garlic, added to pasta sauces and soups, and even used as a "roll-up." They need to be chopped up before cooking unless you are using collard leaves for cannelloni or to make dolmas (stuffed leaves).

***

Kale Chips

Kale is a green, leafy vegetable full of great vitamins and antioxidants, but it ranks poorly among youths. Sautéed with garlic in olive oil with a little salt, kale tastes great, but appreciation for the taste often develops only after age 30 or even 40. Turning kale into chips is a great way of offering a nice familiar crunch. If you like dried seasoned seaweed, you will like this recipe very much.

1 bunch of kale
¼ teaspoon sea salt or garlic salt
1 tablespoon olive oil
1 tablespoon baker's yeast (optional)

Preheat the oven to 350 degrees. Wash the kale and dry it well. Remove thick stems and cut into 2½- to 3-inch strips. Transfer the kale into a plastic bag, add all the ingredients and shake to cover the kale strips evenly. Place on a parchment paper and bake for 15–20 minutes. Enjoy on the same day, otherwise the chips will soften and be not as appetizing.

5. Meats, Poultry, and Seafood

The main course of a dinner is usually a large plate offering a variety of nutritious foods. There should be protein, vegetables, and starch. As many people are trying to lose weight, lower-carbohydrate diets dictate staying away from starches. But the major cause of obesity is truly the overindulgence of refined carbohydrates and fats. Stay away from white breads and non-whole-grain foods. The main-course plate should be divided into two halves. The first half should be brimming with seasonal vegetables and fresh salads. The other half is split between protein and starches. One fourth of your plate is typically 3–5 ounces of your favorite protein, and the other fourth is filled with starches to include brown rice, pilaf, potatoes, couscous, bulgur, or just bread.

The term "protein" encompasses beef, chicken, turkey, lamb, pork, fish, eggs and dairy products, and nonanimal products such as tofu. You can also find a variety of meat substitutes on the market. These foods are vital for rebuilding our tissues and sustaining us on long days. Proteins should comprise about 20% of your total daily caloric intake of nutrients. Here are some suggestions for quick protein courses.

***

Beef

Beef comes from cows. You can purchase it in steak form, ground, or as a roast. People invariably like their beef cooked to different standards. "Rare" means that the beef is very red with only slight graying on the outside, and the internal temperature is 130–140 degrees. Cooking to "medium" gives the meat an internal temperature of 150–160 degrees and a pink color on the inside. Meat that is "well done" is cooked to 160–170 degrees and has no pink left in the middle. The only way that you would know the degree of doneness without cutting into the meat is if you have one of those instant-read food thermometers. Otherwise, you can guess by touching the meat itself. If it seems mushy, then it isn't cooked yet. If, when you press down on the meat, it seems somewhat resistant but still soft, take it off the heat and put it on a plate with foil over it. Once it has cooled to a temperature that you can touch comfortably, slice into the middle. If something needs a little more time on the grill, "touch it up," as I say, and cook the individual slices to the perfection you seek.

Ground beef consists of tougher cuts of meat ground up with varying fat contents. Ground meats can be used in tacos, spaghetti, burgers, chili, meatloaf, and other dishes. As a rule, try to include the leanest meats in your diet.

Hamburgers (per serving)

3–4 ounces lean ground beef
Garlic powder
Salt and pepper
Whole-grain hamburger bun
Lettuce leaves
Thick-sliced tomato
Red onion slices (optional)
Thin sliced pickles (optional)
Optional condiments: mustard, ketchup

Form the ground beef into a ball and gently press it into a patty. Make the patty slightly thinner in the center, as it will expand a small amount. Season the meat lightly with garlic powder, salt, and pepper. Cook the patty either in a broiler, on the stovetop, or on a barbecue grill to your desired doneness. Try not to press down on the burger while it is cooking, as this will squeeze the juices out and leave you with a dry burger.

Place the cooked patty on the hamburger bun and top with lettuce and tomato. If you like, you can add red onions, pickles, mustard, and ketchup.

***

Ground Beef Meatloaf (serves 4)

1 pound lean ground beef
1 slice whole-grain bread, torn into small pieces
1 egg
½ cup finely chopped onion
2 garlic cloves, minced
A pinch each of dried oregano, dried thyme, and dried basil
½ teaspoon each salt and pepper
2 tablespoons ketchup or tomato paste

Place the meat in a bowl. With your hands, mix in the bread, egg, onion, garlic, herbs, salt, and pepper. Don't overmix the meat as it will become hard when cooked. You want it to be pliable and light. Place the meat into a baking dish and form into a round pie shape, about 2 inches high. Spread the ketchup over the top

Bake at 350 degrees for 45 minutes. Slice into wedges and serve. A tossed green salad and cooked corn go well with this meal.

***

Beef Kebabs I

Kebabs originated in Iran and other countries in the Middle East but have become quite popular in the United States. They are a quick and easy way of cooking any cubed or ground meat. "Shish kebab" refers to meat on skewers. It is important to cook the kebabs quickly so they stay moist inside. The ingredients are very similar to meatloaf.

½ cup finely chopped onion
1 tablespoon parsley
1 slice whole-grain bread, dried and turned to crumbs, or softened bread torn into small pieces
1 egg
1 pound lean ground beef (optional: ½ pound ground lamb and ½ pound ground beef)
2 garlic cloves, minced
½ teaspoon each salt and pepper
Pam cooking spray for the baking sheet
Sumac, a dark red Middle Eastern spice available in stores(optional)

Mix onion, parsley, and the bread in a food processor or finely chop them by hand. Add the mixture and the egg to the meat along with the garlic, salt and pepper. Mix well. Take a fistful of mixture, role between your hands into a sausagelike shape, and pat it between your fingers to flatten it. Spray Pam on a baking sheet and place the patties on it. Broil meat 5–6 minutes each side. Serve sprinkled with sumac or without it, with lavash, inside pita pocket bread, or with rice pilaf. You can add tomato, onion, and lettuce into the pocket bread.

***

Beef Kebabs II (per kebab)

4 ounces beef steak, cut into cubes
3 or 4 slices of green, yellow, or red bell pepper, cut into squares
3 mushrooms
3 or 4 thick slices onion, cut into squares
3 or 4 slices of zucchini
Light Vinaigrette
Skewers

In a bowl, mix the meat and vegetables with enough vinaigrette to moisten. Let them marinate for 15 minutes or longer before cooking. Skewers may be metal or wood. If you are using bamboo skewers, they need to be soaked in water for 20 minutes before cooking so they don't burn. Thread the meat and vegetables on the skewers and cook on a BBQ grill or in a broiler until the meat is a desired doneness.

Serve with brown rice or rice pilaf and a large tossed green salad.

***

Ground Beef with Green Beans and Tomatoes

1 onion, finely chopped
2 tablespoons olive or canola oil
1 pound ground beef
1 pound trimmed green beans, cut into 1½-inch tubes
1 (8-ounce) can tomatoes (or 1 cup fresh peeled tomatoes)
½ teaspoon salt
¼ teaspoon pepper (optional)
2 tablespoons finely chopped parsley

Sauté the onions in the oil about 2 minutes., Add the ground beef, and as soon it turns brown, add the washed green beans. Add the tomatoes, salt, and pepper, bring to boil, and simmer for 20–30 minutes. Test the beans for doneness, then turn off the heat and sprinkle with parsley.

Serve with pilaf or brown rice and green salad.

***

Beef with Broccoli and Asparagus over Rice (serves 4)

1 flank steak, about 1 ¼ pounds
1 bunch broccoli, cut into florets
1 small bunch asparagus, trimmed and cut into 2-inch pieces
⅓ cup low-sodium soy sauce
¼ cup white wine vinegar
1 tablespoons sesame oil

2 tablespoon canola oil
1 tablespoon freshly grated ginger
Black pepper
4 cups brown rice, cooked

In a skillet, cook the flank steak on the stove top about 5 minutes per side or until no longer red in the middle. Let cool. Cut the steak in half lengthwise and then into thin slices across the grain. (The lines in the beef are perpendicular to your slicing).

Steam the broccoli until tender. Remove the broccoli and place in a bowl. Using the same water, cook the asparagus until tender. Drain the asparagus and place in the bowl with the broccoli. Add the sliced beef into the vegetables.

Mix together the soy sauce, vinegar, oils, ginger, and pepper in a small bowl. Set aside.

When ready to serve, stir the soy dressing into the flank steak and vegetables. Serve over brown rice. Orange slices are a nice accompaniment to this meal.

***

Grilled Flank Steak with Peppers and Onions (serves 4)

The peppers and onions can be grilled alongside the flank steak, making this is a quick and easy meal. Roast new potatoes in the oven while the meat is cooking and toss a green salad just before serving.

1 flank steak, about 1 ¼ pounds
Olive oil
½ teaspoon ground cumin
½ teaspoon garlic powder
½ teaspoon each salt and pepper
¼ teaspoon cinnamon (optional)
1 red bell pepper
1 yellow bell pepper
1 red onion

Rub the flank steak with a small amount of oil on both sides. Mix together the dried seasonings and rub onto the steak on both sides. Slice the peppers in half and remove the cores. Slice into strips. Remove the onion's papery outer layer and cut the red onion into ½-inch-thick slices. Toss the peppers and onion slices with a small amount of olive oil to moisten. On a preheated grill, place the flank steak, peppers, and onions. If you have a grilling basket, this makes cooking the vegetables easier. Cook the flank steak for 5 minutes on the first side, then turn over and cook to desired doneness. The vegetables should be ready about the same time as the steak.

Slice the steak against the grain and serve with the vegetables alongside.

***

Roasts, such as cross-rib or chuck, are tougher cuts of meat. They are best eaten when slow cooked to tenderize them. If you notice, there are usually very few streaks of fat in the meat. Unless it is tenderloin, little marbling of the meat typically indicates that you will need to slow cook it or tenderize it to keep it from being difficult to chew.

Simple Roast Beef

1 beef round roast, about 5 pounds
Salt and pepper

Preheat your oven to 450 degrees.

Place a metal rack in a roasting pan and place the meat on top of it, fat side up. Generously season the meat with salt and pepper. Add about ¼ inch of water to the bottom of the pan.

Put the roast in the middle of the oven and reduce the baking temperature to 350 degrees. Cooking time will vary between 10 and 20 minutes per pound. To test doneness, insert a thermometer into the roast; 120 degrees is very rare. Cooking to 130 or 140 degrees is about right. Remove the roast from the oven and tent with foil to allow the meat to rest for 15 minutes. Slice thinly and serve. This is great with potatoes, broccoli, and a big salad. Leftover slices may be used in sandwiches, burritos, and egg hash.

**

Chicken

Every whole chicken has two half breasts, two thighs, two drumsticks, two wings, and a back. The thighs, drumsticks, and back consist of darker meat. The breasts and wings are white meat. The dark meat has more robust flavor while the white meat is mild. The darker meat is also moister.

To cut up a chicken, you need to find the joints and slice through them. It is easier than cutting through the bone. You can use heavy-duty kitchen scissors, but a sharp knife that you are comfortable wielding is also good. Starting with the legs, bend the knees and cut through the bend where the softer cartilage is. The same with the wings; slice through where they are attached to the shoulder. Find the thighs by working your fingers up from where you cut the drumsticks off. Feel the joint where the thigh is attached to the back and cut through it. Slice through the ribs on each side to separate the back from the breasts. Finally, slice through the softest part of the breast bone (through the center) and separate the breasts halves. This method works for cooked chicken as well as raw.

**

Roast Whole Chicken (serves 4)

1 whole chicken
Olive oil
Salt, pepper, garlic powder

Preheat oven to 350 degrees.

Remove the wrapping from the chicken and pull the "packaging" out of the chicken cavity. These are the giblets and consist of the liver, gizzard, and heart. I usually discard these, as they tend to be high in cholesterol.

Rub the chicken with a little olive oil and sprinkle salt, pepper, and garlic powder over the skin. Place the chicken in a baking dish breast-side up, tucking the legs and wings underneath, and place it in the oven. Cook for 1 hour. After you take the chicken out of the oven, cover it with foil and let it rest for about 10 minutes before you carve into it. This helps juices reabsorb. Cut your chicken into pieces, or slice the breast as one does with the Thanksgiving turkey.

Leftover chicken can be removed from the bone with your fingers and used in burritos, enchiladas, sandwiches, and salads.

***

Basic Baked Chicken Pieces

Your choice of a chicken breast, thigh, or leg, skin on
Salt, pepper, and your choice of dried herbs, such as thyme or basil, or a combination of several

In a small baking dish, place your chicken skin side up. Sprinkle with seasonings and bake in a 350-degree oven for 25 minutes, or until there is no longer any pink in the center of the chicken piece. Larger pieces will take longer to cook.

Remove chicken from oven and cover with foil for about 5 minutes before serving.

***

Asian Chicken Salad with Bok Choy and Cucumber (serves 2)

1 boneless, skinless chicken breast half
Salt and pepper
3 cilantro sprigs plus 3 tablespoons chopped cilantro
½ whole green onion, plus 1 green onion, chopped
¼ pound sugar snap peas

2 baby bok choy, thinly sliced crosswise
½ English cucumber, quartered lengthwise, then thinly sliced crosswise
2 tablespoons soy sauce
1 tablespoon seasoned rice vinegar (or a touch more)
1 tablespoon canola oil
2 teaspoons peeled and minced fresh ginger

Poach the chicken breast by bringing a medium skillet filled with
water and a pinch of salt to a boil. Add the chicken breast, 3 cilantro
sprigs, and whole green onion. Reduce heat to simmer and poach
chicken until cooked through. If you need to, cut the chicken breast in
half to make sure it is no longer pink in the middle. Transfer chicken
to a platter to cool. In the same water, cook the sugar snap peas until
crisp-tender, about 1 minute.

Drain and cool the sugar snap peas, discarding the whole green
onion and cilantro sprigs. Coarsely shred the chicken. Mix chicken,
chopped cilantro, chopped green onions, snap peas, bok choy, and
cucumber in a bowl. Whisk together soy sauce, vinegar, oil, and ginger in a bowl. Add dressing to the chicken mix and toss to coat. Season with salt and pepper.

***

Sweet and Savory Chicken Breasts (1 serving)

This recipe is easily multiplied for company.

1 small half chicken breast, skin on
½ ounce goat cheese, or a goat cheese and light cream cheese
mixture
1 tablespoon hot pepper jelly
Salt and pepper

Preheat the oven to 350 degrees.
Using your fingers, loosen the skin on the chicken and form a

pocket. Place the cheese in the pocket and press down to spread it out over the meat. Brush the pepper jelly over the skin and bake for 35 minutes.

The chicken skin is a conduit for moistening meat and holding the cheese onto the breast. Avoid eating it, however, as it is loaded with saturated fats, which none of us needs.

Note: If you wish to wow friends, you can place fresh sage leaves over the cheese under the skin in a decorative pattern before baking.

***

Chicken Parmigiana (per serving)

One chicken breast, flattened with the palm of your hand
½ teaspoon Italian herbs
½ cup marinara sauce, from a jar
Shredded Parmesan cheese

Preheat oven to 350 degrees.

Place the chicken breast in a small baking dish and sprinkle with the herbs. Spoon marinara sauce over and sprinkle with a generous amount of Parmesan cheese. Bake for 25–30 minutes or until chicken is no longer pink in the middle. This is delicious served with noodles, Caesar or tossed green salad, and a steamed vegetable.

***

Grilled Chicken Sandwich

The chicken for these sandwiches may be made ahead and reheated in a slow oven just before serving.

1 small boneless chicken breast, flattened
Salt, pepper, paprika, garlic powder
Slice of Havarti or jack cheese (optional)

Hamburger roll or toasted sourdough bread
Lettuce, tomato, sliced red onion, sliced avocado
Dijon mustard

Cut the chicken breast in half so that you have 2 thinner pieces. Using the palm of your hand, press down on the chicken pieces until somewhat flattened. Season with the spices andplace on a BBQ grill or cook in a 350 degree oven until no longer pink inside, about 15 minutes or so . If you add the cheese, place it on the chicken just about a minute before removing from heat. It should be melted.

Serve the chicken breast on the bread of your choice and add condiments.

***

Chicken Sausages with Cannellini Beans (serves 4)

Chicken sausages are widely available at most grocery stores. Look for the ones that come from free-range chickens. Those are usually precooked and need only 4–5 minutes of heating.

1 clove garlic
2 tablespoons olive oil
1 can cut tomatoes with or without herbs
1 15-ounce can cannellini beans
1 package chicken sausages (4–5)

Add the garlic once the olive oil is heated in the pan, then add the tomatoes and the white beans. Heat for about 7–8 minutes until it starts to boil. Heat the sausages per package instructions, cut them into 3–4 slices each, and add to the pan; cook with tomato-bean mixture without mixing for another 5 minutes. Serve over rice or with potatoes. This recipe goes really well with lamb-sherry sausages. You may find those in fancy stores or some farmer's markets.

***

Lamb

Lamb can be pricey, particularly if you go with delicate lamb chops, but ground lamb is not as expensive. Mixing ground lamb with other meats such as ground beef or ground turkey can provide a great flavor. You can also grill lamb shoulders or any other cuts of lamb. Leg of lamb may be purchased quite reasonably at discount warehouse stores such as Costco.

***

Grilled Lamb Chops

Though expensive, this recipe is very easy to follow and always turns out great.

½ teaspoon salt
¼ teaspoon pepper
6 lamb chops

Sprinkle the salt and pepper evenly on the lamb chops and grill on a lightly greased rack over a hot flame 5-6 minutes a side.
Serve with pilaf and green salad of your choice.

***

Roast Leg of Lamb

Fresh garlic
1 leg of lamb, butterflied
Salt and pepper

Mince several cloves of garlic and rub over the roast. Season with salt and pepper and cook on a BBQ grill or broil in the oven to desired doneness, about 15 minutes each side. Lamb is as delicious rare as it is cooked to well-done. It is your personal choice how much to cook the meat.

After cooking, remove from heat and cover with foil for about 10 minutes before slicing the meat.

Roast lamb is delicious by itself served alongside roasted vegetables, spinach or tossed green salads, and new potatoes or brown rice. The sliced lamb also makes a delicious sandwich served on toasted rolls or pita bread with caramelized onions and other condiments of your choice.

***

Pork

Pork refers to the meat of pigs. It comes in roasts, ground, and smoked, such as in bacon. Pork should never be eaten raw. To safely cook pork, the meat should reach an internal temperature of 160 degrees. "Quick read" meat thermometers are a great way to test the temperature of your meats. Broiling, grilling, stove-top cooking, slow cooking, and roasting are all good methods to use when cooking pork.

Pork bacon should be eaten rarely, and only that which has been processed without nitrites or nitrates. These are preservatives. Along with the smoking seasoning and salts, these are not good foods for you!

The pork tenderloin is a long strip of tender pork that usually weighs just over a pound. They can usually be purchased in vacuum-sealed packaging with two tenderloins. Use one now and freeze the other for later.

***

Grilled Pork Tenderloin (serves 4)

1 pork tenderloin
Olive oil or canola oil
Salt, pepper, garlic powder

Start your BBQ and bring the temperature up to 350 degrees. Alternately, you can broil or bake this small roast. Remove the outer white filmy thin skin and tendons from the tenderloin using a sharp knife. Rub some oil over the lean meat and season it with the salt, pepper, and garlic powder. Place the tenderloin on the grill and close the lid. Cook for 10 minutes. Open the cover and turn the pork over. Cook for another 5–7 minutes or so, until the center is just barely pink. Remove from the heat onto a platter and tent the meat with foil.

After the meat has cooled slightly, cut the meat into ½-inch slices. Serve on plates and drizzle with the juices on the platter. Roasted new potatoes, a large green salad, and steamed broccoli or cauliflower are great complements to this meal. Leftover pork works well for sandwiches, burritos, or by itself for another supper.

***

Pork Cutlet Stir-Fry (per serving)

Canola oil
Fresh finely grated ginger, about 1½ teaspoons
1 large clove garlic, minced
4 ounces pork cutlet, cut into strips
1 small baby bok choy, chopped
1 carrot, sliced
1 celery stalk, sliced
½ bell pepper (any color), cut into strips
Soy sauce

In a skillet or a wok, heat a tablespoon of oil over medium heat and add the ginger and garlic. After about 30 seconds, add the pork and cook, stirring frequently, until it is no longer pink. Remove the meat from the pan and set aside.

Add another small amount of oil to the same pan and cook the vegetables until they are just tender. Add the reserved pork back to the pan and stir it into the vegetables. Season with soy sauce and serve over rice.

***

Pork Loin Roast

Pork loin is typically an inexpensive cut of meat. Learning how to cook these roasts will save money and time, as you can use the leftovers for subsequent meals for dinner or in sandwiches, burritos, or whatever you can think of.

1 small pork loin, about 2 pounds
Salt, pepper, dash of garlic powder, and a pinch of dried rosemary and thyme

Preheat an oven to 350 degrees. Season the pork loin with the salt, pepper, garlic powder and herbs, and place in a small baking pan, fat side up. Bake for about an hour, or until a thermometer inserted in the roast reads 155 degrees.   Remove from oven and tent the meat with foil for about 15 minutes before slicing. Leftover pork roast slices make great sandwiches.

***

Turkey

Guacamole Burgers *(enough guacamole for 2 people)*
This is just your basic burger topped with fresh guacamole. Enjoy!

Guacamole:
1 avocado, slightly soft but not mushy
1 lemon wedge
Salt, pepper, garlic powder
1 slice of Sonoma jack or Swiss cheese
Turkey burgers, consisting of a grilled 3- to 4-ounce burger with melted cheese, buns, lettuce and other condiments

Remove the pit and skin from the avocado and place it in a bowl. Mash it with a fork and squeeze lemon juice into it so it doesn't turn brown. Season with salt and pepper and a small dash of garlic powder. Pile a big spoonful on top of your burger. Yum!

***

Turkey Meatloaf

1 package ground turkey (1¼ pounds)
1 slice of bread, torn into small pieces
1 egg
½ cup chopped onion
½ cup chopped walnuts
6 mushrooms, chopped
Canola oil
Dijon mustard

Using your hands, mix together the meat, bread pieces, egg, onion, walnuts, and mushrooms in a bowl. Don't overmix or the turkey may become too firm and dry. Pat the mixture into a small loaf pan. Alternately, you may pat this into a round shape and place in a baking dish. Spread a small amount of canola oil over the top of the meat and then spread with Dijon mustard.

Bake in a 350-degree oven for 40 minutes. Cut into ½-inch slices and serve.

***

Asian Turkey Burgers (serves 4)

1 package ground turkey
1 can water chestnuts, drained and chopped
4 scallions, chopped
¼ cup chopped cilantro, plus extra sprigs for serving
2 cloves garlic, minced
1 tablespoon finely shredded fresh ginger
2 tablespoons soy sauce

½ teaspoon black pepper, or ½ teaspoon red pepper flakes
1 tablespoon canola oil or Pam spray
Sesame seeds
Fresh lettuce leaves, such as green or red leaf
Kaiser rolls

Using your hands, mix ground turkey, chopped water chestnuts, chopped scallions, chopped cilantro, minced garlic, shredded ginger, soy sauce, and seasonings together in a bowl. Add a small amount of water to the mix if it seems dry. Don't overmix. Form four patties with the meat mixture. Patties may be made up to 8 hours in advance and kept chilled.

Spray your BBQ grill with Pam or rub with oil. Cook the patties over medium heat, turning once, for 10–12 minutes. You may also broil these in the oven.

Sprinkle the cooked patties with sesame seeds and serve on rolls with a couple lettuce leaves and additional cilantro sprigs. A tossed green salad with mandarin oranges, scallions, and sliced almonds is a great complement to this meal.

***

Fish and Shellfish

Offering seafood these days is a delicate balance for suppliers. With environmental disasters and overfishing, our supply of good-quality seafood has become limited. Sadly, this also means that it has become expensive. However, it does matter where you buy the fish. Frozen fish is readily available in most supermarkets. It's mostly wild caught and instantly frozen, so it is the best quality. Most fish is high in omega-3 fatty acids and is easy and fast to cook. Salmon, sea bass, tilapia, red snapper, flounder, Dover sole, mahi mahi, and ahi tuna, among others, are good choices.

Fish tastes great broiled, baked, grilled, or poached. Remember, fish cooks fast and it's easy to overcook. Make sure you have lemons when you plan to cook fish. Lemon and fish love each other.

Most people like salmon. Of the differing species, chinook and sockeye have a higher fatty content, which means a higher amount of valuable omega-3 fatty acids. Defrost the fish overnight in the refrigerator. Open the plastic container and pat dry the defrosted fish.

Occasionally you will encounter a "fishy" smell. If your fish is fresh but overly fragrant, simply soak the fillets in milk for about 15 minutes before preparing to cook.

***

Poached Salmon with Dry Tarragon and Asparagus

Dill will also work well with this dish.

½ cup water, or more
½ cup white wine
½ onion, sliced
1 tablespoon dried tarragon
¼ teaspoon paprika
1 salmon fillet, 4-5 ounces
10 spears trimmed asparagus

Bring the water, wine, onion, herb, and paprika to boil in a large skillet. Add the salmon skin-side down and cook for 5–7 minutes until it all turns pink. Take the salmon out and add the asparagus for another 5 minutes. Remove the skin and serve the salmon on one side of the plate with rice and asparagus on the other.

***

Broiled Salmon Fillet (1 serving)

This simple preparation of salmon provides a standard by which you can cook other oily fishes as well. Alternate toppings may be used, such as fruit salsas or herb dressings, but the basic lemon wedge squeezed over top is best to bring out the delicious flavor of a wild-caught salmon.

1 (4-ounce) salmon fillet (salmon steaks are okay, too)
1 teaspoon olive oil to brush over (optional)
Salt and pepper
Lemon wedges

Set oven temperature to broil. Place the salmon, skin side down, on a piece of foil on a pan suitable for broiling. If using olive oil, brush over the fish and then season lightly with salt and pepper. Cook until fish flakes at thickest part when prodded with a fork. For a ½- to 1-inch-thick fillet that is about 3 inches from the heat source, the cooking time is about 5–10 minutes, and you don't need to turn the fish. The skin often sticks to the foil, so this makes for easy cleanup. Carefully lift up the salmon, leaving the skin behind. Plate the salmon and serve with lemon wedges.

You can use the same foil technique for the outdoor barbecue. Place your salmon skin-side down on a piece of foil. Brush with a small amount of olive oil, squeeze lemon juice over the fish, and season with salt and pepper. You may use other herbs or spices as you wish. Fold up the foil around the fish and seal it to enclose the fish. Place on a hot barbecue grill and cook for about 5–7 minutes. Wait until it cools slightly before opening the foil packet. The skin usually sticks to the foil, so use a gentle hand when lifting the salmon and you will get a skinless fillet. Enjoy your salmon!

***

Salmon or Trout with Vegetables (serves 2)

2 large tomatoes, sliced
1 onion, sliced
1 bay leaf
Salt and pepper

1 green or red bell pepper
2 salmon fillets, 4 ounces each

Cook the tomatoes, onion, bay leaf, salt, pepper, and bell pepper for 10 minutes until soft. Nestle the salmon slices inside the liquid, cover, and cook for 5–7 minutes. Turn the heat off and discard the bay leaf. Serve with mashed potatoes.

***

Oven-Poached Fish, Franciscan Style

This recipe is modified from the cookbook of the Franciscan Crab Restaurant on Fisherman's Wharf in San Francisco.

8 new red potatoes or fingerlings, cut in half
Large handful of cubed butternut squash or baby carrots
½ teaspoon salt
¼ teaspoon pepper
1 teaspoon fresh rosemary
2 garlic cloves, left whole but papery skin removed
Olive oil
2 fish fillets (sea bass, mahi mahi, Dover sole, flounder, tilapia, or any other white fish)
Lemon juice from ½ lemon
4 spears asparagus
Handful of sliced olives (optional)

Place the potatoes, cubed squash or carrots, salt, pepper, rosemary, and garlic cloves into a baking dish. Drizzle with olive oil and bake for 25 minutes at 375 degrees. Rub the fish with olive oil, lemon juice, and a pinch of salt. Nestle it onto the potato mixture and top with asparagus and olives. Continue cooking for another 8–10 minutes. Serve in a baking dish (colorful dishes are quite inexpensive at Marshall's and Cost Plus) with a large green salad.

***

White Fish with Lemon Zest and Butter (serves 2)

1 tablespoon butter, softened
Zest from ½ lemon
Pinch of salt and dash of pepper
4 small fish fillets, 4 ounces each

Heat a nonstick skillet to hot. Mix the butter, lemon zest, salt, and pepper and rub it on the fish. Place the fillets on the hot skillet and cook for 5 minutes until one side is browned. Turn and cook the other side. It takes 3–4 minutes to finish cooking.

This fish can be used for fish tacos or eaten with mashed potatoes and steamed vegetables.

***

Mahi-Mahi in Asian Marinade

This recipe can be used for any fish, including tilapia, swai, or cod.

¼ cup soy sauce
2 teaspoons sesame oil
2 tablespoons honey
2 slices fresh ginger root
2 cloves garlic crushed
1 lemon, squeezed
Salt and pepper to taste
2 tablespoons olive oil
2 to 3 fillets, 4 ounces each

Mix all the ingredients, except for ½ tablespoon of olive oil in a bowl and marinate fish for half an hour to 1 hour. Heat the pan, add the olive oil, and pan-fry the fillets 4–5 minutes on each side until a crust is formed, turning only once. Serve with rice and vegetables.

***

Prawns and Shrimp

Prawns, shrimp, clams, mussels, scallops, lobster, and crab are part of the shellfish family. They are bottom feeders, so one has to be careful when buying them that they come from cleaner waters. They are readily found frozen and fresh. You need to remove the shell before eating. When cooking the bivalves, make sure they open when steaming. Discard those that don't open up.

Prawn and Vegetable Kebabs (per serving)

4 large prawns or shrimp
Red pepper, cut into 1-inch squares
Zucchini, cut into ¼-inch slices
Red onion, cut into 1-inch squares
Mushrooms (optional)
Light vinaigrette, or just olive oil and vinegar with salt and pepper
1 large skewer

Light up the barbecue.
Remove the shell body but leave the tail on the prawns. In a bowl, toss the prawns and vegetables together with vinaigrette to moisten. Thread the prawns and vegetables on the skewer, alternating the pieces. Grill until the prawns about 3 minutes and turn over. Cook another 3 minutes or so until the prawns are pink all the way through and the vegetables are tender. This is great served over brown rice and with a large green salad.

***

6. Starches and Grains

Here are some simple recipes to go with the main course and vegetables. This group comprises rice and other grains and seeds, potatoes, pasta and noodles, beans, and legumes.

***

Basic Baked Potato

1 potato, skin scrubbed under running water to remove dirt
Olive oil
1 tablespoon light sour cream or plain yogurt
I tablespoon salsa
½ ounce shredded cheddar or Parmesan cheese (optional)

Preheat oven to 350 degrees. Poke a sharp knife into center of potato (this slit will let air escape during baking and keep the potato from exploding in your oven). Rub a little olive oil over the skin. Place on baking rack in the oven and cook for about 1 hour, or until the potato is cooked. A cooked potato "gives" when squeezed. Slice the potato halfway through and open it up. Top with a dollop of light sour cream or plain yogurt, your favorite salsa, or a sprinkling of cheddar or Parmesan cheese. Avoid the butter, as it adds unnecessary calories from fat and cholesterol.

***

Half-Baked Potatoes

1 potato per person
Olive oil
Coarse salt and pepper

Scrub potato and slice it in half lengthwise. Place cut side up in a baking dish and drizzle with olive oil. Season with salt and pepper. Bake for an hour at 350 degrees. The potato halves should be puffed with a golden crust on top.

***

Roasted Potatoes

3 cups organic potatoes, scrubbed clean and cut into ½-inch cubes
1 cup baby carrots, cut into half
2 tablespoons olive oil
1 teaspoon rosemary
½ teaspoon salt
¼ teaspoon pepper

Mix the vegetables in a roasting pan and toss with the olive oil and seasonings. Bake for 35–40 minutes at 350 degrees, turning veggies over with a spatula about halfway through.

***

Red, White, and Blue Potatoes (serves 4)

1 pound red, white, and blue new potatoes of similar size, scrubbed
3 scallions chopped, or 2 tablespoons diced red onion
¼ cup chopped parsley
¼ cup crumbled blue cheese
Light Vinaigrette (see Salad Dressings)
Salt and pepper to taste

Cook the new potatoes in gently boiling water until tender, about 15 minutes. Let them cool and then cut them into pieces all about the same size. Place the potatoes in a bowl along with the scallions, parsley, and blue cheese. Gently toss the potato salad with enough vinaigrette to moisten the potatoes. Season to taste if needed.

***

Caesar Potato Salad (serves 6 or more)

This recipe combines our beloved Caesar salad with new potatoes for a hearty side dish.

1 recipe for Caesar salad, no dressing added
1 pound new potatoes, cut into quarters
Caesar salad dressing, See chapter 3
Extra lemon, Parmesan cheese, if needed

Place ingredients for the Caesar salad (lettuce, croutons, and parmesan) in a large bowl. Cook the potatoes until tender and let cool until they are comfortable to handle. Cut them into halves or quarters, and add to the salad ingredients in the bowl. Toss with the dressing. Squeeze lemon over and add more Parmesan if needed.

***

Rice

Rice is a relatively inexpensive grain and can be eaten by itself or mixed into salads. White rice is a refined product. Milling and polishing of white rice results in the loss of 90% of its B vitamins, and a similar loss of other vital nutrients. For that reason we recommend the use of brown rice, wild rice, or unrefined rice.

Rice is very easy to cook. You just need a saucepan with a lid. For 1 serving: Place ½ cup of rice in the pan. Add about 1 cup of water. The water-to-rice ratio when cooking is typically 2:1. Occasionally, when making moister rice like arborio (risotto) or sticky rice, more liquid may be required. Bring the water and rice to a boil over high heat on the stove. Reduce the heat to a simmer, stir, and cover the saucepan with the lid. Different rices have different cooking times. Check the package of your rice to see how long to cook it. When cooking brown rice, the water-to-rice proportion changes to 2½:1. Brown rice takes about 35–45 minutes. If you soak the brown rice overnight, it cooks as fast as the white rice.

***

Seasoned Rice

This is also good when you add to the sauté mixture chopped carrots, scallions, mushrooms, peas, or any other herb or vegetable that you have on hand.

¼ cup chopped onion
1 tablespoon olive oil
1 clove garlic, finely chopped
1 cup cooked brown rice

Sauté onion in olive oil for about 3 minutes. Add garlic and cook an additional 30 seconds. When onion is softened, add rice and stir until heated through. A small amount of chicken broth may be added if the mixture seems dry.

***

Rice Pilaf

Rice pilaf is very popular among people who originated from the Middle East. Just like pasta in Italy, pilaf is eaten daily, but you don't need to eat anything daily with the variety of foods available to you. You can use white rice or brown rice to make pilaf. White rice should be soaked for 30 minutes if it is round rice; soaking is not needed if it's long grain. Brown rice should be soaked overnight or at least for 3 hours; that makes it much easier to cook.

2 nests curly, fine vermicelli
2 tablespoons butter, canola oil, or olive oil
2 cups chicken broth, vegetable broth, or water, boiling (use 2½ cups liquid if you're using brown rice)
1 cup rice
½ teaspoon salt if you are using water (might not be needed if you're using broth, which already has salt added to it)

Break up the vermicelli with your hands and stir it in the oil on low heat until golden. Add the boiling water or broth and the rice, stir to mix, and simmer on low to moderate heat, 15–20 minutes for white rice or 30 minutes for brown rice. Let stand for 5 minutes before serving. Add salt if needed.

***

Coconut Rice

When cooking 2 cups of rice, add 1 can light coconut milk in place of equal parts water. Cook until rice is tender. Just before serving, stir in ½ cup finely chopped scallions and ¼ cup flaked and sweetened coconut.

***

Wild Rice Salad with Apricots (serves 4)

2 cups wild rice, cooked
⅓ cup dried apricots, chopped into ¼-inch pieces
¼ cup scallions, chopped
¼ cup slivered almonds
Light vinaigrette
Salt and pepper to taste

Mix all ingredients in a bowl and toss with enough vinaigrette to moisten the salad. Season to taste.

Note: Wild rice salads may be made using any combination of fruits and nuts. Try mixing wild rice with dried cranberries, toasted pecans, scallions, and even blue cheese.

***

Rice and Fruit Salad (serves 6)

Olive oil
1 apple, cored and cut into ¼-inch cubes
1 small red onion, cut into ¼-inch cubes
1 stalk celery, cut into ¼-inch cubes
1 small carrot, peeled and cut into ¼-inch cubes
1 clove garlic, minced
3–4 cups wild rice, cooked
2 tablespoon apple cider vinegar
3 tablespoons balsamic vinegar
1 tablespoon fresh lemon juice
½ cup slivered almonds, toasted
2 tablespoons currants
1 teaspoon coarse salt
Pepper

In a skillet, heat 2 tablespoons olive oil and cook the apple, red onion, celery, carrot, and garlic until the onion is transluscent, about 5 minutes. Transfer to a bowl with the wild rice and add the currants.

Return the skillet to the heat and add the vinegars and lemon juice. Whisk constantly until some of the liquid evaporates and the amount is reduced by half (to about 3 tablespoons total). Add in 2 tablespoons olive oil and whisk until blended. Drizzle dressing over the rice and vegetables and mix thoroughly. Season to taste with salt and pepper. Serve chilled or at room temperature with the toasted almonds on top.

***

Polenta

Polenta is made of coarsely ground bits of degerminated corn. It is featured in Italian cooking and here in America. It can be soft like porridge or cooked hard and sliced. Either way, it is a versatile low-fat food that can substitute for pasta and potatoes as part of a meal, and it is super simple to prepare.

Firm polenta slices can be used in place of noodles in lasagna, and it can be served with your favorite sauces or stews on top, such as chili or beef stew. Firm polenta may also be grilled and served as a side dish. Softer polenta can also be served as a side dish instead of mashed potatoes and as a base for other condiments, just like the firmer polenta.

Basic Firm Polenta (serves 8)

3 cups water
Pinch of salt
2 cups polenta, or corn grits
1-2 tablespoons butter or olive oil
¼ cup grated Parmesan cheese

Bring a pot of water to boil and add the salt. Gradually stir in the polenta using a long-handled wooden spoon. Reduce the stove heat to medium-low and let the polenta simmer gently for about a half hour, stirring occasionally to break up lumps and keep it creamy. Also, make sure it doesn't burn on the bottom. Stir in the butter or oil.

Meanwhile, oil a small baking dish. When the polenta is cooked, spoon it into the prepared dish and let it set for about 15 minutes. Cut the polenta into squares and serve hot with Parmesan cheese sprinkled over.

***

Creamy Seasoned Polenta (serves 2–3)

2 cups chicken stock
1 clove garlic, minced
½ cup yellow cornmeal
¼ cup grated Parmesan cheese, plus extra for sprinkling over
2 tablespoons olive oil
Salt and black pepper

Heat the chicken stock in a saucepan. Add the garlic and cook over medium-high heat until the stock comes to a boil. Reduce the heat to medium-low and slowly add the cornmeal, stirring constantly with a wooden spoon. Simmer for 7–10 minutes, stirring constantly, until thick. Remove the polenta from the heat and stir in the ¼ cup of Parmesan cheese, olive oil, ½ teaspoon of salt, and pepper. Stir until smooth and serve hot, sprinkled with extra Parmesan cheese.

7. Pasta and Noodle Main Dishes

"Everything you see I owe to spaghetti."

Sophia Loren

Pasta is the simplest and fastest to prepare among all foods. It is the national Italian dish that is enjoyed all over the world. With the low-carbohydrate boom, many people who are trying to lose weight are shying away from pasta. But, remember, no weight gain comes from a particular food. It comes from overeating those foods. Many Italians eat pasta every single day, but they are not overweight as a nation. For college students, pasta, with its easy recipes, huge variety, and room for imagination, is probably the simplest and most economical meal you can make. And who doesn't like pasta?

The first secret for success in making good pasta is to cook it in a large pot. Most pastas typically double in volume when they are cooked. You need to bring a 4- to 6-quart pot of water to a boil and add a tablespoon of coarse salt. Salted boiling water is a beginning to every pasta. Then you carefully read the instructions and add the pasta. It is a good idea to stir the pasta once or twice during cooking so the pasta doesn't stick together. Typically any pasta will cook in 8–10 minutes after it starts boiling, so always time the pasta cooking. You can test one piece or strand to see if it meets your standards. You don't want pasta that is crunchy, which means that it is undercooked. If it is overcooked, it will be mushy. Somewhere in between there is perfect. *Al dente* ("firm to the bite") is your best result. Drain the pasta in a colander and do not rinse with warm water. If you talk to Italians and real pasta pundits, they recommend against rinsing the pasta with water. If you cook your pasta exactly according to the package, you do not need to rinse it. You can even use some of the drained pasta water to moisten the noodles if you wish. Once pasta is cooked, it's ready to get sauced!

By the way, don't be intimidated by the variety of names for the pastas. They are merely describing the shapes of the noodles. Angel hair is very fine spaghetti, linguine and fettuccine are thicker and flatter, penne is tubular, ziti is a thick long tube, orzo looks like big grains of rice, orechiette looks like little ears, farfalle is like butterflies, and lasagna is wide and flat. Also, more and more we are seeing whole grain pastas. They are nuttier in flavor and have a denser texture, which means they will fill you up while eating less. Whole-wheat and whole-grain pastas are loaded with more protein and fiber than the white variety, so that is even more reason to get used to using them.

Every pasta recipe follows three basic steps:
- Boil the pasta in salted water and drain.
- Prepare the sauce.
- Mix the first two and top it with cheese before serving.

To garnish the pasta you can use chopped parsley. You will see that a lot of pasta has red crushed pepper or black pepper added. That is completely optional. Italians like it a little spicy—*picante*. Italians will tell you that you have to use certain pastas with certain sauces, but as a college student you can use any pasta you have with any of the sauces.

As for cheeses, the most frequently used is Parmesan cheese, which you can buy already grated or grate yourself. Other cheeses, such as gorgonzola, mozzarella, ricotta, feta, soft sheep's cheeses, and goat cheeses, may also be used in the sauces. Once you make your own pasta sauce, you will realize which ingredients are tastier and add more of them when you make it another time.

Start with a large bowl of salad and the pasta of your choice and it will be a full entree. Here comes the million-dollar question: what is the serving size for pasta? The most commonly accepted serving size is 2 ounces of uncooked pasta or 1 cup of cooked pasta. To refresh your memory, 16 ounces is equal to 1 pound of pasta. Leftover pasta should be eaten within a day or two.

***

Simple Tomato and Basil Pasta (serves 4)

1 (8-ounce) package angel hair or penne pasta
3 tablespoons olive oil
2 cloves garlic, minced
2 cups Roma (plum) tomatoes, diced, or 1 can of peeled tomatoes
Crushed red pepper to taste
Freshly ground black pepper to taste
2 tablespoons chopped fresh basil or 1 teaspoon dried basil
¼ cup grated Parmesan cheese

Bring a large pot of lightly salted water to a boil. Add pasta and cook for 8 minutes or until al dente; drain. Pour olive oil in a large, deep skillet over high heat. Sauté the garlic until lightly browned and then discard it. Reduce heat to medium-high, add tomatoes, and simmer for about 8 minutes. Stir in red pepper, black pepper, and basil; simmer for another 3–5 minutes. Add cooked pasta, tossing thoroughly with sauce. Serve topped with grated Parmesan cheese.

***

Pasta with Marinara Sauce (serves 8) (vegetarian/vegan)

This is similar to the previous recipe. If you don't have time to make this sauce, just buy a jar of marinara and pour over your cooked pasta!

2 tablespoon olive oil
3 cloves minced garlic, or ½ teaspoon garlic powder
1 (28-ounce) can tomatoes, undrained and chopped
1 teaspoon sugar
¾ teaspoon salt

½ teaspoon pepper
¼ cup fresh basil, chopped
¼ cup fresh parsley, chopped
16 ounces cooked spaghetti
Parmesan cheese (optional)

Heat oil in a large saucepan over medium heat. Add garlic and cook about 1 minute, stirring constantly. Add tomatoes, sugar, salt, and pepper and bring to a boil. Reduce the heat and simmer for ½ hour, occasionally stirring. Add in the basil and parsley and cook for another minute. Serve over the pasta. Sprinkle optional Parmesan over the pasta. This sauce can be frozen.

Calories for one serving of pasta sauce, 2 ounces of whole-grain spaghetti, and a large tossed green salad.

***

Pasta with Meat Sauce (serves 8)

Olive oil
1 small onion, diced
1½ pounds ground beef or ground turkey
Salt and pepper
Marinara sauce from previous recipe, or 2 jars of marinara sauce
1 pound cooked spaghetti
Parmesan cheese, grated

Heat a tablespoon of olive oil in a large skillet and add the onion. Cook and stir the onion for a few minutes until it is softened. Add the meat and break it up with a spoon. Cook until no more pink shows in the meat. Add salt and pepper to taste. If there is excess oil or grease in the pan, scoop it out and discard it. Add the marinara sauce and stir into the meat and onion mixture. Season the sauce to taste with salt and pepper. Serve over the hot cooked pasta and top with optional Parmesan cheese. Serve with a large tossed green salad.

***

Pasta with Meatballs (serves 4)

For meatballs:
1 pound lean ground beef
1 large egg, beaten
¼ cup bread crumbs or ½ slice stale bread, soaked in a small amount of milk and crumbled
1 tablespoon Romano grated cheese
1 tablespoon minced fresh parsley
1 large clove garlic, minced fine
½ teaspoon salt
Pepper to taste

For pasta:
Marinara sauce
16 ounces spaghetti, penne, or other pasta
Finely chopped basil and basil leaves
2 tablespoons Parmesan cheese

Mix the ingredients for meatballs until well blended. Form meatballs and place in baking pan with a little cooking oil. Bake at 375 degrees for 15 minutes. You may also cook the meatballs over a medium heat in olive oil until golden, about 10 minutes. Add the meatballs to heated marinara sauce, mix well, and simmer for 10 more minutes. Meanwhile, cook the pasta according to the package, drain, and mix with the sauce. Sprinkle with chopped basil and Parmesan cheese, and garnish with basil leaves.

***

Pasta with Pesto (serves 4)

Purchase pesto at the market. You will find it in the refrigerator section with fresh pasta, or in the freezer section. Sometimes you can also find it canned in glass jars.

8 ounces cooked whole-grain pasta
½ cup pesto
Grated Parmesan cheese

Cook the pasta according to package directions and drain in a colander, reserving a couple of tablespoons of the cooking liquid. Return the pasta to the pot and bring it to boil. Turn the heat off and add the ½ cup of pesto sauce to the pot, tossing to coat the pasta well. Remove the mixture to a large bowl. Stir in the Parmesan cheese until well blended.

Making pesto is time consuming, but if you have lots of basil and want to try making it yourself, you can try the following recipe. This sauce comes together quickly in a blender or food processor.

2 large bunches of fresh washed basil leaves, or about 4 cups
2 tablespoons pine nuts
½ cup extra virgin olive oil
¼ teaspoon salt
2 garlic clove, peeled
½ cup Parmesan cheese

Combine the basil, pine nuts, olive oil, salt and garlic in the blender and process until it is finely minced. Add in the Parmesan cheese and blend until combined.

***

Chicken with Pesto Pasta (serves 8)

1 (16-ounce) package bow-tie or penne pasta
1 tablespoon olive oil
1 clove garlic, minced
2 boneless, skinless chicken breasts, cut into bite-size pieces
Crushed red pepper flakes to taste
⅓ cup oil-packed sun-dried tomatoes, drained and cut into strips
½ cup pesto sauce

Cook the pasta according to the package directions. Heat the oil in a large skillet over medium heat. Sauté garlic until tender, then stir in chicken. Season with red pepper flakes. Cook until chicken is golden and cooked through. In a large bowl, combine pasta, chicken, sundried tomatoes, and pesto. Toss to coat evenly.

***

Tuna and Tomato Pasta (serves 4)

1 (8-ounce) package angel hair or penne pasta
3 tablespoons olive oil
2 cloves garlic, minced
2 cups Roma (plum) tomatoes, diced, or 1 can of peeled tomatoes
Crushed red pepper to taste
Freshly ground black pepper to taste
1 can (7 ounces) of solid white tuna in olive oil
¼ cup grated Parmesan cheese
1 tablespoon flat-leaf parsley, chopped

Cook the pasta according to the instructions until al dente; drain. Pour olive oil in a large, deep skillet over high heat. Sauté the garlic until lightly browned and then discard it. Reduce heat to medium-high, add tomatoes, and simmer for about 8 minutes. Stir in red pepper, black pepper, and the tuna; simmer for another 2–3 minutes. Add cooked pasta, tossing thoroughly with sauce. Serve topped with grated Parmesan cheese. Garnish with parsley.

***

Pasta with Pears and Gorgonzola (serves 4)

2 ripe pears
2 tablespoon butter
1 teaspoon lemon juice
1 cup crumbled gorgonzola

8 ounces pasta (penne, rigatoni, ziti)
1 tablespoon finely chopped walnuts
1 tablespoon flat-leaf parsley, chopped

Core the pears and slice them ¼-inch thick. Saute the chopped pears in butter and lemon juice for 5 minutes on low-medium heat, then add the gorgonzola cheese. Cook the pasta according to directions. Leave a little bit of water in the pot. Add the pear sauce and serve sprinkled with the walnuts and flat-leaf parsley.

***

Cold Pasta with Mozzarella Cheese (serves 8)

16 ounces penne pasta
2 tablespoons olive oil
2 minced garlic cloves
1 28-ounce can organic peeled canned tomatoes
Pinch of red and black pepper to taste
2 tablespoons chopped fresh basil
1 cup cubed mozzarella cheese
1 tablespoon finely cut basil leaves and 3 whole basil leaves

Bring a large pot of lightly salted water to a boil. Add pasta and cook for 8 minutes or until al dente; drain and let it cool. You can add a teaspoon of olive oil to help keep the pasta from sticking together. Cut tomatoes into cubes, add the minced garlic, olive oil, salt, pepper and chopped fresh basil. Add the cubes of mozzarella cheese to the cold sauce and refrigerate for an hour. Add the cold sauce to the cooked pasta and toss it thoroughly. Serve cold, garnished with basil leaves. This pasta is great in the summer.

***

Pasta and Grilled Vegetable Salad (serves 6)

Any combination of grilled vegetables may be used in pasta salads. Cut all the vegetables into similar size pieces. This recipe has an Italian flair.

1 eggplant, cut into ½-inch-thick slices
Salt and pepper
1 zucchini, quartered lengthwise and cut into ½-inch-thick slices
1 red bell pepper, seeded and chopped
½ red onion, chopped
Light vinaigrette
6 cups hot cooked Israeli couscous or orzo pasta
½ cup (at least) chopped fresh basil
Olive oil

Place eggplant in a colander and sprinkle with ¾ teaspoon salt. Toss gently to coat. Let stand in the sink or on a plate for about ½ hour. Rinse with cold water and drain well.

Lightly oil or spray a grill rack for the barbecue. Toss the eggplant, zucchini, bell pepper, and red onions with about a tablespoon of light vinaigrette in a bowl, then grill for about 15 minutes, turning once. Remove from grill and let cool. Add the grilled vegetables to the hot pasta along with basil leaves. Toss with vinaigrette to moisten the salad and season to taste with salt and pepper. More olive oil may be added to the salad if needed.

***

Orzo and Shrimp Salad (4 servings)

2 cups cooked orzo
1 cup frozen peas, thawed
½ cup finely chopped red onion
A handful of chopped fresh parsley

1 pound medium-sized cooked shrimp, peeled
Italian Herb Vinaigrette (see dressings)

Add orzo, peas, onion, parsley, and shrimp to a large bowl. Toss with Italian Herb Vinaigrette to moisten and flavor the dish. Chill until ready to serve. Toss again and check the seasonings before serving.

***

Tortellini Salad (serves 6)

1 (9-ounce) package fresh cheese tortellini, cooked
1 small head broccoli, cut into florets
1 pint cherry or grape tomatoes
1 avocado, peeled and cut into ½-inch cubes
1 jar oil-packed artichoke hearts, cut in quarters (optional)
4 scallions, sliced
Herbed buttermilk dressing or ranch dressing

Place pasta and vegetables together in a large bowl. Toss with just enough dressing to moisten the salad. You may add artichoke marinade from the jar to add extra juice to the dish. Chill until ready to serve.

***

Stuffed Pasta Shells (serves 6-8 persons per baking dish)

After the shells are stuffed and before they are baked, they may be frozen. This recipe makes enough to fill two 9x13-inch baking dishes.

1¼ pounds ground turkey
1 large onion, chopped
1 egg, stirred with a fork
¾ cup grated Parmesan cheese, divided
1 cup ricotta cheese

2 cups shredded mozzarella
¼ cup dry bread crumbs, or 1 piece toasted bread torn into small pieces
1 teaspoon dried Italian seasoning (a mixture of dried oregano and basil works fine)
2 jars marinara sauce
1 package jumbo pasta shells, cooked and drained

Preheat the oven to 350 degrees. Sauté the meat in a skillet over medium heat until no pink shows. Drain the meat and set it aside in a large bowl. Sauté onion in the same skillet until soft. Add the cooked turkey, onion, egg, ½ cup of the Parmesan cheese, ricotta cheese, mozzarella cheese, bread crumbs, and seasoning to the cooked meat. Mix all together well.

Spoon about ½ cup sauce in the bottom of each baking dish. Fill each of the cooked shells with some of the meat mixture and place in the baking dishes. Pour the rest of the sauce over the pasta shells and sprinkle with remaining ¼ cup of the Parmesan. Bake for 25-30 minutes. Serve with a large green salad tossed with a light vinaigrette.

***

Pasta with Arugula and Shrimp (serves 4)

2 cloves garlic, peeled and chopped
¼ cup olive oil
12 uncooked shrimp, shells off
2 tablespoons white wine
1 cup washed, drained arugula (optional)
8 ounces farfalle, penne, or rigatoni
¼ teaspoon red pepper flakes (optional)

Sauté chopped garlic in olive oil for 1 minute. Do not allow garlic to brown. Add the raw shrimp and white wine and cook until shrimp are fully cooked and pink. Add the arugula and cook for another minute. Cook the pasta according to directions, drain, and place in a bowl. Add the sauce, mix thoroughly, and sprinkle with red pepper flakes if desired.

***

Spaghetti with Arugula and Smoked Salmon (serves 4)

1 clove garlic, chopped
2 tablespoons olive oil
1 cup washed, drained arugula
4 ounces smoked salmon, cut into stripes
8 ounces spaghetti
Pinch of red pepper flakes (optional)
1 tablespoon capers

Sauté chopped garlic in olive oil for 1 minute. Do not allow garlic to brown. Add the arugula and the salmon and cook for another minute, constantly stirring.

Cook the pasta according to directions, drain, and place in a bowl. Add the sauce and optional red pepper flakes if desired, mix thoroughly, and sprinkle with capers.

***

Seafood Pasta (serves 4)

1 tablespoon olive oil
½ small onion, chopped
1 large clove garlic, minced
1 jar marinara sauce
1 teaspoon dried Italian seasonings (or a mix of dried basil, thyme, and oregano)
1-pound package frozen mixed seafood, such as calamari, shrimp, and scallops
8 ounces cooked whole-grain linguine or spaghetti
Grated Parmesan cheese

Heat the olive oil in a skillet over medium low heat and cook the onion and garlic until soft. Add the marinara sauce and seasonings and simmer for about 5 minutes. Add the seafood and cook for another 3 minutes or until the shrimp are pink. (Plan on adding the seafood just before you are ready to serve—if you overcook it, it tends to get tough.) Serve on pasta with Parmesan sprinkled over.

***

Broccoli with Elbow Pasta (serves 8)

3 medium-sized broccoli florets
2 tablespoons olive oil
2 garlic cloves
16 ounces pasta of your choice, although elbow, penne, and fusilli work particularly well
Freshly ground pepper and salt
Crushed red pepper flakes
4 tablespoons grated Parmesan cheese

In a large pot of boiling water, blanch broccoli for about 5 minutes. You can also just steam the broccoli. Drain, and set aside. Heat olive oil in a large skillet over medium heat. Sauté garlic until lightly golden, then discard it. Add the broccoli and sauté, stirring occasionally, for about 10 minutes. Broccoli should be tender yet crisp to the bite.

Meanwhile, cook the pasta in a large pot of boiling salted water according to instructions or until al dente. Drain, and place in a large serving bowl. Toss with the broccoli, and season with salt, pepper, and hot pepper flakes. Serve with Parmesan cheese.

***

Noodles

Noodles originated in Asia. Most cultures have noodles as a part of their cuisine. These days you can find a Thai or Vietnamese noodle house on the same street as an Italian pasta shop.

Traditionally noodles are made from wheat (udon and ramen) or buckwheat (soba). You can also find noodles made from rice (white and brown), mung beans (cellophane noodles or Chinese vermicelli), and even acorns (Korean). They are used in soups, salads, and main dishes, and served hot or cold. Noodles are typically cooked in broth or water, but some noodles merely need to be soaked before using. Most noodles will have a recipe on the packaging. Some come already with the spices that you need to use which makes the recipe much easier.

Ramen noodle soups are readily available and are very inexpensive. When buying these soups, make sure they do not contain partially hydrogenated oils and MSG (monosodium glutamate). MSG is a great preservative and flavor enhancer and is used in many Asian canned and preserved foods. It is safe to eat it on occasion, but if you're eating those soups daily or several times a week, try to avoid MSG.

Vegetable Chow Mein (serves 4)

½ pound fresh noodles
1 can water chestnuts
½ red bell pepper
1 cup fresh snow peas
2 celery stalks
2 slices ginger
2 tablespoons oil for stir-frying, or as needed
1 cup mung bean sprouts
2 tablespoons soy sauce
Pinch of sugar

Blanch the noodles in boiling water for 3–5 minutes, or cook according to the package directions. Prepare the vegetables: Rinse all the vegetables and drain thoroughly. (Rinse canned water chestnuts under warm running water for several minutes to remove any tinny taste). Cut the red bell pepper in half, remove the seeds, and cut into thin strips. String the snow peas, and cut the celery into thin strips on the diagonal. Mince the ginger. Heat the wok and add 2 tablespoons oil. When the oil is hot, add the minced ginger and stir-fry briefly until aromatic. Add the water chestnuts. Stir-fry briefly, and add the other vegetables except for the mung bean sprouts. Stir-fry briefly and add the noodles. Stir in the soy sauce and sugar. Stir in the bean sprouts. Cook for a few more seconds and serve.

***

8. Stir-Fries

Stir-frying is normally associated with Asian cooking, but it's an easy way of cooking any vegetables and meats. It makes a fast main-course dish that is amenable to good imagination and creativity. You need a wok or large skillet, thinly sliced vegetables or meats, and sauces to moisten the cooking food. As a rule you'll need the following ingredients to start a stir-fry:

- Garlic
- Ginger
- Soy sauce
- Sesame oil
- Canned sliced chestnuts (optional)
- Green onions
- Cilantro or parsley
- Sweet peas
- A wok

***

Tofu Stir-Fry (serves 4)

4 tablespoons vegetable oil
2 cloves garlic, chopped
4 tablespoons soy sauce
4 tablespoons rice vinegar
1 tablespoon Thai chili sauce

8 ounces extra-firm tofu, cut into ¼-inch cubes
1 tablespoon sesame oil
8 ounces bean sprouts
8 ounces shredded carrots
1 green bell pepper, thinly sliced
8 green onions, halved lengthwise

Heat the vegetable oil in a wok over medium-high heat; cook and stir the garlic until lightly browned, about 2 minutes. Pour in the soy sauce, rice vinegar, and chili sauce; stir to mix, then bring the mixture to a simmer. Reduce heat to medium-low and let the sauce simmer for 10 minutes. Transfer the sauce to a bowl, and stir the tofu into the sauce. Set the tofu mixture aside.

Heat the sesame oil in the same wok; cook and stir the bean sprouts, carrots, green pepper, and green onions until the vegetables are bright in color and slightly wilted, about 5 minutes. Pour in the tofu with sauce; stir to combine. Serve over rice or pasta.

***

Beef and Vegetable Stir-Fry (serves 4)

1 teaspoon minced ginger
1 teaspoon minced garlic
1½ cups sliced mushrooms
1 pound steak, cut into 2-inch-long, thin slices
1 cup snow peas
¾ cup green onions, sliced
¼ cup soy sauce
2 teaspoons chili sauce
1 teaspoon chopped cilantro

Heat the oil in a large nonstick skillet, then add the garlic, ginger, and mushrooms. Stir-fry until mushrooms are tender, about 3–4 minutes. Add the beef and cook until beef is brown, another 3 minutes.

Add the snow peas, ½ cup of the green onions, the soy sauce, and the chili sauce. Saute until peas are crisp. Serve with rice or noodles. Sprinkle with remaining green onions and cilantro.

***

Chicken Stir-Fry (serves 4)

1 pound chicken breasts
Canola oil
2 carrots, sliced
2 stalks celery, sliced
Fresh mushrooms, quartered
1 cup fresh sweet peas
1 small bag bamboo shoots
1 medium onion, cut into chunks
1 medium green bell pepper, cut into chunks
1 medium zucchini, cut into slices
½ small bottle Kikkoman stir-fry sauce

Cook the chicken separately, then slice it and set it aside. Heat canola oil in wok, and add carrots and celery. Stir-fry, and when they are starting to get a little tender, add the rest of the vegetables and the chicken. Stir-fry until vegetables are crisp-tender. Add Kikkoman stir-fry sauce; simmer for a few minutes. Serve over white or fried rice.

9. Pizza

Why would you make your own pizza when it is so easy to purchase one that is already made? The reason is simple: it allows you to control the salt, fat and carbohydrate content and can be much healthier. Making your own pizza follows three main steps, just as pasta does: make or buy the crust, pile on the sauce and toppings, and bake it. The fun part is that you can use a variety of toppings and omit any topping you are not fond of. The good news is that if you're making a pizza with a friend or two, each one can pick a corner and place his or her own favorite toppings.

Basic Boboli Cheese Pizza (makes 1 pizza to serve 4 people)

One large Boboli thin-crust pizza
Olive oil
1 cup pizza sauce or marinara sauce
2 ounces grated part-skim mozzarella
2 ounces grated mild cheddar
2 ounces grated jack cheese
Sprinkling of Parmesan cheese

Brush the pizza pie with olive oil. Spoon the sauce over and sprinkle the cheeses evenly over the sauce. Bake according to package directions, until the cheese is melted.

Add a large tossed green salad with light vinaigrette and you have a whole meal.

If you like a variety of flavors on your pizza, you may add additional toppings such as vegetables and meats. For the above recipe, after brushing with olive oil and spreading with sauce, sprinkle only half the cheese over. Layer your choice of toppings on top of the cheese. When you are satisfied, sprinkle the rest of the cheese over all. Bake on a cookie sheet until the cheese is melted and the crust is golden.

Some stores sell fresh pizza dough. It comes in a variety of flavors and types, such as whole grain or whole wheat, and herb. Sprinkle your countertop with flour and roll out the dough to the desired size. Use a bottle if you don't have a rolling pin. You can use a cookie sheet to bake the pizza; just roll the dough into a rectangle shape. Spray your baking sheet with Pam and place the pizza dough on it. Brush a little olive oil on the dough and add toppings. Bake according to the dough package instructions.

Optional topping ideas: a small can of sliced black olives, drained; sliced mushrooms; sliced tomato; sliced onion; sliced bell peppers; anchovies; canned pineapple, drained and chopped; artichoke hearts; fresh herbs, such as basil, cilantro, thyme, and marjoram; ½ pound cooked extra-lean sausage, crumbled; leftover BBQ chicken, shredded; low-fat pepperoni or salami slices; or anything else that sounds good.

Here are a few tried-and-true, good flavor combinations for your pizza:

- Olive oil, marinara sauce, fresh basil leaves, Parmesan, and mozzarella cheese—this is a Margherita pizza.
- Mexican Pizza: olive oil, tomato sauce, leftover taco meat, shredded cheddar cheese, sliced onions, sliced and drained olives. If you like more heat, diced jalapeno peppers may be sprinkled over before baking. To cool this down, serve with sour cream and guacamole or chopped avocado.
- Basic Combo Pizza: Olive oil, marinara sauce, shredded mozzarella and Parmesan cheeses, cooked Italian sausage, sliced pepperoni and salami, sliced red and green peppers, sliced red onion, optional sliced olives.
- BLT Pizza: Olive oil, tomato sauce, crumbled cooked bacon, tomato slices, mozzarella and cheddar cheese. After cooking, sprinkle

shredded lettuce over or just serve a salad on the side. In Brazil, they break eggs onto their pizzas before cooking. The oven cooks them wonderfully and it adds a new twist to the pizza.

- Garlicky Clam Pizza: Liberally brush pesto sauce over your dough instead of olive oil. Add a layer of shredded mozzarella, Parmesan cheese, 3 cans drained clams, 4 cloves of fresh minced garlic, a whole bunch of parsley chopped up, more mozzarella, and a drizzle of olive oil over the top.
- Potato Pizza: You probably have never seen this type of pizza unless you've been to Italy. Cover the pizza dough or the ready crust with olive oil and then with very thinly sliced potatoes. Sprinkle with salt and rosemary, and cover with another layer of olive oil.

10. Soups

"Let me be the first to tell you that drinking alcohol is the worst thing you can do in cold weather. Hot soup is the best because the process of digesting food helps to warm you up."

Morgan Freeman

These days, a variety of healthy canned or boxed soups is available in most stores. When you don't have time to make a batch of homemade soup, you can always count on organic brands such as Amy's, Eden, or others. Lentil and bean soups are hearty meals and will provide you with lots of fiber and protein. Stick with broth-based soups and avoid soups made with heavy cream, such as bisques or chowders, if you are worried about calories. (Manhattan clam chowder is a red- broth-based exception, while the New England clam chowder is a cream-style variety). A simple lunch or dinner might consist of a bowl of soup, side salad or vegetable, and a whole-grain roll. Believe it or not, this is really all you need to eat!

As a college student, a can of soup, a whole-grain roll, and an apple should be an easy and affordable meal. The following homemade soup recipes are designed to be affordable and will provide you with several meals.

Onion Soup with Cheesy Topping (serves 6)

4 tablespoons olive oil
4 onions, thinly sliced
1 tablespoon flour
½ teaspoon pepper
2 quarts of beef broth
Thick slice of French bread for each bowl of soup
Grated gruyere or Swiss cheese
Grated Parmesan cheese

Heat olive oil in a heavy saucepan over medium-high heat. Add the onion and sauté over medium-low heat until golden, about 20–30 minutes. Stir in the flour and season with the pepper. Reduce the heat and add the broth. Simmer over low heat for about 20 minutes.

Preheat your broiler. Lightly toast the French bread slices. Transfer soup to heatproof serving bowls. (A heatproof bowl is one that may be Pyrex or ceramic, certified by the label on the bottom of the container). Place the toasted bread on top of the soup and top with a generous helping of gruyere or Swiss cheese and then a sprinkling of Parmesan cheese. Place under the broiler until cheese is bubbly. Serve immediately.

***

Easy Chicken Noodle Soup (serves 8)

1 whole chicken, inside pouch and loose giblets discarded
16 cups water
2 tablespoons chicken bouillon seasoning made with no partially hydrogenated fats and no MSG
2 stalks celery with leaves, cut into small pieces
2 carrots, peeled and cut
1 whole onion, chopped
1 bay leaf, and a pinch of other spices that you like, such as basil, marjoram, rosemary, and thyme

1 pound package noodles (whole-grain angel hair or spaghetti), cooked

In a large stockpot, place the whole chicken in with the water and bring to a simmer. Skim off the fat after it has collected on the surface. Add the boullion, celery, carrots, onion, and desired seasonings. Cover the pot with a lid and simmer for 1½ hours. Remove the pot from the heat and let cool. The broth will be reheated and used later, so don't toss it down the sink!

When cool enough to handle, take the chicken out of the pot and remove the skin and bones. With your hands, shred the chicken into large pieces and set aside.

When ready to serve, place some cooked warm noodles in the bottom of a bowl, add some of the shredded chicken, and ladle the reserved and reheated broth over.

Saving the leftovers: place the chicken in a zip-top bag, the noodles in a different bag, and the broth in a different container. By storing the components of the soup separately, the noodles and chicken won't get mushy.

***

Miso Soup (serves 6)

Miso soup is a traditional Japanese soup made out of the stock called dashi, miso paste, small cubes of tofu, and other optional ingredients. Most dashi is made from a mixture of shaved fish and kelp. Dashi granules can be purchased in most Asian supermarkets. To make the stock, mix ½ teaspoon of dashi with 1 cup of water.

2 teaspoons dashi granules
4 cups water
3 tablespoons miso paste
1 (8-ounce) package silken tofu, diced
2 green onions, sliced diagonally into ½-inch pieces

In a medium saucepan over medium-high heat, combine dashi granules and water; bring to a boil. Reduce heat to medium and whisk in the miso paste. Stir in tofu. Separate the layers of the green onions, and add them to the soup. Simmer gently for 2–3 minutes before serving.

***

Vegetable Miso Soup

5 cups stock made out of dashi
1 ounce dried shiitake mushrooms
½ pound firm tofu, cut into ¼-inch cubes
1 sheet nori, cut into thin strips
2 teaspoons fresh grated ginger
1½ cups small broccoli florets
¾ cup grated carrots
4 tablespoons white miso
Green onions, thinly sliced

In a large soup pot, bring the stock to a boil. Remove from the heat and add the dried mushrooms. Cover and let stand for about 15 minutes or until the mushrooms are softened. Remove the mushrooms from the broth and remove and discard their stems. Thinly slice the mushroom tops and set aside.

Add the tofu, nori, and ginger to the broth. Bring the soup to a simmer and cook for 3 minutes. Add the mushrooms, broccoli, and carrots and simmer for another minute.

Remove 1 cup of the soup and add the miso to it. Stir the cup of soup and miso until the miso is dissolved. Add the dissolved miso broth back to the large pot of soup. Serve the soup immediately. (Once the miso has been added, it is best not to reboil the soup). Garnish with green onions.

***

Minestrone (serves 4)

Minestrone is a soup made with a variety of fresh vegetables and simmered in broth. Make sure you wash all vegetables first. A cup of cooked noodles or a can of drained beans may be added as well.

2 tablespoons olive oil
½ onion, diced
1 leek, white part only, thinly sliced
1 carrot, peeled and thinly sliced
1 stalk celery, thinly sliced
1 garlic clove, minced
3 unpeeled tomatoes, seeded and chopped
½ green cabbage, coarsely chopped
½ pound fresh green beans, ends trimmed and cut into ½-inch pieces
2 quarts chicken stock
1 bunch spinach or 1 bunch kale, coarsely chopped
Pepper
¼ cup Parmesan cheese, grated

In a large soup pot, heat the oil and add the onion, leek, carrot, celery, garlic, tomatoes, cabbage, and green beans. Sauté the vegetables for 3–5 minutes, stirring often. Add the stock and bring the soup to a boil. Lower the heat and simmer, uncovered, for 25 minutes. Add the spinach or kale and cook for 5 minutes more. Taste the finished soup and adjust the seasonings by adding pepper. Serve the soup and sprinkle 1 tablespoon Parmesan cheese over.

***

Vegetable Soup (serves 4)

This French-style soup is thickened with the vegetables, not cream.
2 tablespoons canola oil
1 large onion, chopped

1 large leek, white part only, sliced
3 cans (14 ounces each) chicken broth
1 medium-size potato, peeled and diced
1 medium-size turnip, peeled and diced
8 carrots, thinly sliced
¼ teaspoon thyme leaves
Salt
Additional broth, if needed

In a soup pot, heat the oil and add the onion and leek. Cook, stirring the vegetables, until they are soft. Add the broth, potato, turnip, carrots, and thyme. Bring to a boil. Cover the pan, reduce the heat, and simmer until the vegetables are very soft (about 20 minutes).

Puree the mixture in a blender or food processor and return to pan. Be careful not to burn yourself with the hot soup. Season with salt to taste. Thin with additional broth if desired.

***

Lentil Soup (serves 8)

There are three commonly occurring lentils: brown, French green, and red. For this soup you can use brown or French green lentils.

2 cups lentils
½ teaspoon each salt, pepper, paprika
1 onion, finely chopped
1 carrot, chopped
1 celery root, chopped
2 tablespoons olive oil
Parsley for garnish

Wash the lentils well and cook in 4 cups of water for 30 minutes, until tender. Add salt, pepper, and paprika to the boiling water. Sauté onions, carrots, and celery root in olive oil about 5 minutes. Add the cooked lentils with the liquid; simmer for 20 minutes. Add salt and pepper to taste. When serving in bowls, sprinkle chopped parsley over.

***

11. Herbs

Leafy herbs are a great addition to any dish. Conveniently, herbs are often dried and you can use them when a fresh bunch is not available. The following is a quick list of popular herbs and ways to use them.

- Basil: a great addition to Italian food, also as a topping or condiment for Asian food, it can be added to fresh green salads, pastas, used to make sauces such as pesto, in spring rolls, in noodle dishes, etc.
- Cilantro; popular in Asian and Hispanic cultures, it is used in salsas, salads, soups, in spring rolls, in noodles dishes, and in sauces.
- Mint: most international cuisines use mint, whether it be in sauces, jellies, teas, spring rolls, fresh green or fruit salads, or desserts.
- Oregano: found in cuisines throughout the Mediterranean and Middle East as well as South America, it pairs well with basil in sauces and other foods, and in marinades for meats.
- Parsley: common in the Americas, Europe, and Asia, it comes in two different varieties, flat leaf and curly leaf. Parsley is used fresh in salads, such as green salads or grain salads like tabbouleh, sprinkled over soups and stews, in sauces, as a garnish, and in seasoning blends such as gremolata (lemon zest, olive oil, and parsley). Parsley has a vibrant taste and bright green color and in Europe is used as a garnish to every meal, including pasta, soup, potatoes, meats, salads, antipasto, and many other foods.

12. Dessert

Dessert is a special treat, and the occasional desserts are fun to make, serve, and eat. Of course, no one can deny the heavenly smell that fresh baked cookies impart to our homes!

Fruits are the basis of a variety of great finishes to your meal. A fruit salad is easy to prepare and can be made in advance. Sorbets are frozen ices, similar to ice cream but without the cream. Fruit compote is cooked and can be served warm or cold. Fruit pies are easy to make. You can buy a premade crust and follow the recipe on the box for fillings and cooking. All desserts are high in calories, so rule number one is to stick to one serving size and don't eat dessert every single day.

***

Brownies with Walnuts

Brownies have dozens of recipes and always turn out great. The main ingredients are natural and simple and usually include sugar, eggs, cocoa, flour, and oil or butter. Walnuts are optional; if you don't have any, just omit the walnuts. Brownies certainly qualify to be an Alpha Plan food, but because of their richness they should be eaten in small amounts.

½ cup vegetable oil or 1 stick unsalted butter
1 cup sugar
1 teaspoon vanilla extract

2 eggs
½ cup unbleached all-purpose flour
½ cup unsweetened cocoa powder
¼ teaspoon baking powder
¼ teaspoon salt
½ cup chopped walnuts

Preheat oven to 350 degrees. Grease a 9x9-inch baking pan. In a medium bowl, mix together the oil (if you are using butter, cut into ¼-inch pieces and melt), sugar, and vanilla. Beat in eggs. In another bowl, combine flour, cocoa, baking powder, and salt; gradually stir into the egg mixture until well blended. Stir in walnuts, if desired. Spread the batter evenly into the prepared pan. Bake for 20–25 minutes, or until the brownies begin to pull away from the edges of the pan. Let cool on a wire rack before cutting into squares. Brownies can be made a day or two ahead and could be stored airtight at room temperature.

***

Berries and Cream (½ cup berries per serving)

Blueberries
Strawberries
Raspberries
Blackberries

Good-quality vanilla yogurt, sweetened with honey or sugar if needed
Mix all berries together. Place berries in a serving bowl and top with a generous dollop of sweet yogurt. Garnish with mint.

***

Tropical Fruit Salad (serves 4)

This simple salad is very sweet. A little bit goes a long way. Try adding it to your yogurt.

1 papaya, peeled and cut into ½-inch cubes
1 cup pineapple, cut into cubes
1 mango, peeled and cut into cubes
About ½ inch of finely grated fresh ginger, or ¼ teaspoon almond extract
1 tablespoon unsweetened (organic) shredded coconut

Toss the papaya, pineapple, and mango together with the fresh ginger or a drop of almond extract. Sprinkle the coconut over just before serving.

***

Ice Cream!

Everyone likes ice cream, right? These days there are so many flavors we couldn't dare to name them all. One thing you have to look for, though, is added "junk." Stay away from ice creams that have high fructose corn syrup, artificial flavors and colors, and partially hydrogenated products in them. Good old-fashioned ice cream, made with real milk and cream and real flavorings and extracts, is what you want to consume.

For a fun dessert, add toppings to your scoop of ice cream. Chocolate chips, nuts, chopped fruit, and jam are just a few of the many ways to dress up your dessert.

***

Apple Pie

1 purchased pastry crust
4 or 5 Granny Smith or other tart apple, peeled, cored, seeded
½ cup sugar
1 teaspoon cinnamon
Pinch of ground nutmeg
Pinch of ground mace
2 tablespoons butter
Preheat oven to 375 degrees.

Roll out the dough if you need to and place in a pie pan. Thinly slice the apples and pile into prepared crust. Sprinkle with sugar, cinnamon, nutmeg, and mace. Cut the butter into small pieces and evenly distribute them over the apples and spices.

Bake for 45 minutes so that the apples are bubbling and the crust is golden. Remove from the oven and let cool. Serve with vanilla ice cream and/or hot coffee.

13. Party favorites

Parties are a lot less expensive when you make some of the food yourself. Ask guests to bring their favorite appetizer or even a meat dish or a side dish. Here are some easy recipes that can be made for large crowds.

***

Hummus (Aunt Dora's)

Hummus is a popular Middle Eastern dish made out chick peas, or garbanzo beans. These days it's also very easy to find hummus in any store. However, it's a lot cheaper when you make it, particularly for a big party. Also, most hummus sold in the markets contains some sort of preservative. Hummus can be served as an appetizer with pocket bread, crackers, carrots, celery, cucumbers, or fresh bell peppers. It always comes out well and preserves really well for at least a week. To make it from scratch, you need a food processor or a blender. Canned chick peas are available at every supermarket and also in organic forms. For a crowd of 30, multiply the recipe by four.

1 (15-ounce) can chick peas, drained, but not dried (save a teaspoon of the liquid from the can)
1 lemon, squeezed
1 tablespoon tahini (sesame seed paste, available in most supermarkets)
1 clove garlic

Pinch of salt
1–1½ tablespoons olive oil

Combine all in the Cuisinart and process to paste. Hummus made out of 1 can of chick peas is the perfect amount for a small Cuisinart. Once you're making it, it makes sense to make more than 1 can, so just repeat the recipe. Sprinkle with olive oil and garnish with a black olive, thinly sliced carrots and/or parsley. Serve in a shallow dish and combine with pita bread and vegetables. This dish is universally loved and is as vegan as it gets, so your vegan friends would appreciate it.

***

Seven-Layer Vegetarian Dip

1 (16-ounce) can refried beans
4 cups shredded cheddar-Monterey jack cheese blend
1 (8-ounce) container sour cream
1 cup guacamole
1 cup salsa
1 (2¼-ounce) can black olives, chopped
½ cup chopped tomatoes
½ cup chopped green onions

Spread the beans into the bottom of a serving tray that is about 1½ inches deep. Sprinkle 2 cups of shredded cheese on top of beans. The sour cream is spread over the cheese and then the guacamole goes on top of the sour cream. Pour salsa over guacamole and spread evenly. Sprinkle remaining shredded cheese on guacamole. Sprinkle black olives, tomatoes, and green onions on top. You can serve this dish immediately, or refrigerate it overnight and serve cold. I think it tastes better at room temperature. Serve with corn chips. Note: A layer of ground beef seasoned with taco flavors can be also added.

***

Antipasto Platter

"Antipasto" means "before the meal" and is comparable to hors d'oeuvres. Simply arrange a variety of meats and cheeses on a plate, accompanied by marinated vegetables, olives, and some breadsticks. This appetizer offers a colorful presentation, and guests can pick and choose what they would like to try. The following suggestions may be found at most grocery stores or Trader Joe's:

½ pound salami
¼ pound sopressata (Italian cured, dry salami)
½ pound prosciutto (thinly sliced Italian ham)
½ pound sliced provolone
Marinated mozzarella balls
Large jar of marinated artichoke hearts, drained
Large jar of pickled vegetable (giardiniera) salad, drained
Marinated large olives, also available in bulk in stores
Jar of roasted red peppers, drained and cut into pieces
Hard-boiled eggs, cut into quarters (optional)
Carrot and celery sticks (optional)
Baguette slices and breadsticks

Arrange the meats and cheeses on a plate or cutting board. Put the vegetables in bowls around the meats. Place the breads in a basket next to the arrangement. Place small forks out next to the meats and cheeses and into the vegetable bowls to serve. Also, put an empty bowl out for olive pits if needed.

***

Crab Ceviche with Peppers

Ceviche, or seviche, is a raw fish marinated in citrus and chili peppers that is popular in Central and South America. This recipe, though, uses cooked and canned crab meat.

12 ounces fresh crab meat or canned crab meat from the refrigerated section

⅔ cup fresh lemon juice
2 large, fresh diced tomatoes
3 tablespoons fresh chopped cilantro
2 finely chopped garlic cloves
1 diced green bell pepper
1 diced yellow bell pepper
1 diced red bell pepper
½ chili pepper, diced
1 tablespoon olive oil
Salt and pepper to taste

Mix all the ingredients in a bowl. Chill for 1 hour and serve with corn chips.

***

Homemade Chili

Chili is great for a large party. You need a large pot this party-size chili dish.

4 (15-ounce) cans kidney beans, rinsed and drained
2 tablespoons olive oil
1½ cups chopped onions
2 garlic cloves
1 diced green bell pepper
3 tablespoons chili powder
1 pound ground turkey and ½ pound ground beef (meat is optional)
2 (12-ounce) cans chopped tomatoes
2 tablespoons tomato paste
3 cups chicken broth
Chopped fresh parsley

Heat the oil in a large pot. Add the onions, the garlic, and the peppers; stir in the chili powder and the ground meats. Cook until golden brown. Add the rest of the ingredients except the parsley and cook for 45 minutes to an hour. Add salt and pepper to taste. Serve with chopped fresh parsley. Optional toppings may include chopped red onion, shredded cheese, and a dollop of sour cream.

***

Party Chicken, Asian Style (allow 2 thighs per serving)

Asian marinade (see the section on fish, chapter 5) can be used to marinate chicken, fish, or tofu. Fish and tofu are gentler and do not require marinating more than 60 minutes. Chicken, on the other hand, may be marinated overnight.

Asian marinade, freshly prepared
Boneless, skinless chicken thighs

Make the Asian marinade recipe in this book by adding all the ingredients to a bowl and mixing well until smooth. Add the chicken thighs. Marinate the chicken thighs in the refrigerator for at least 60 minutes or overnight. When ready to cook, line a baking dish or cookie sheet with foil and spray with Pam cooking spray. Lay the thighs on the foil and bake at 350 degrees for about 20–45 minutes (depending on the size of thighs) or until cooked through.

***

Fun Menu Ideas for Entertaining

The following menus contain suggestions that are easy to prepare and have recipes in the previous chapters. When having people over for a meal or just for movies and snacks, remember to keep preparation simple so that you, the host, can enjoy yourself.

Antipasto Platter
Spaghetti with Marinara or Meat Sauce
Large Tossed Green Salad with Light Vinaigrette
Purchased ice cream in cones for dessert

***

Seven Layer Vegetarian Dip with Chips
Taco bar with taco shells, seasoned meat, shredded lettuce,
shredded cheese, chopped tomatoes and onions, chopped cilantro,
salsas, and sour cream
Mexican Cabbage Slaw
Sliced watermelon

***

Homemade popcorn
Grilled Chicken Sandwiches
Hummus plate
Tossed Green Salad with Light Vinaigrette
Pasta salad of your choice
Scoop of ice cream

***

Sushi
Asian Marinated Chicken Thighs
CoconutRice
Tossed green salad with mandarin oranges, sliced almonds, scallions light vinaigrette, and sesame seeds

Epilogue

There are an infinite amount of recipes available on the internet, from the very simple to the very complex. With this inexhaustible library at your disposal, try to challenge yourself and your taste buds with new recipes. And remember: food is your friend. It is an instrument of the greatest pleasure and entertainment. However, you must remain thoughtful about it.

Healthy eating in college and beyond will save you a lot of trouble, be it medical conditions, doctors' visits, pill-taking or bill-paying. And please, do not forget to exercise!

Glossary of Acronyms

AHA ---------- American Heart Association
AIDS ---------- acquired immune deficiency syndrome
ALA ---------- alpha-linolenic acid (an omega-3 fatty acid)
AS ---------- artificial sweeteners
BMI ---------- Body Mass Index
BMR ---------- Basic Metabolic Rate
DHA ---------- docosahexaenoic acid   (an omega-3 fatty acid)
DNA ---------- deoxyribonucleic acid
DRI ---------- Dietary Reference Intake
EPA ---------- eicosapentaenoic acid (an omega-3 fatty acid)
FC ---------- food coloring
FDA ---------- U. S. Food and Drug Administration
GI ---------- Glycemic Index
GLP-1 ---------- glucagon-like peptide-1 (an appetite affecting hormone)
HDL ---------- high-density lipoprotein (good cholesterol)
HFCS ---------- high fructose corn syrup
HIV ---------- human immunodeficiency virus
LDL ---------- low-density lipoprotein (bad cholesterol)
MSG ---------- monosodium glutamate
MUFA ---------- monosaturated fatty acids
OP ---------- organophosphorus
PKU ---------- phenylketonuria
RDA ---------- Recommended Dietary Allowance
WC ---------- Waist Circumference

About the Authors

Mariam Manoukian and Kim Fielding live in the San Francisco Bay Area. Together, they ran a medical weight loss clinic based on the Alpha Plan concepts.

Mariam Avakian Manoukian attended the Yerevan Medical Institute in Soviet Armenia, completed postdoctoral training at the All Union Institute of Endocrinology in Moscow. After moving to the United States, she completed her residency at the Santa Clara Valley Medical Center in San Jose, California. She is board certified in internal medicine. She is currently in private practice with her husband, Dr. Jerry Manoukian, and they have two children in high school, ready to start college. Dr. Mariam Manoukian specializes in the prevention and treatment of diabetes and obesity. Her first book, *the ABCs of Diabetes* was published in 1990 in Armenia. In 2005, she and her husband coauthored the *Metabolic Syndrome Survival Guide*, dedicated to lifestyle changes necessary to avoid diabetes.

Kimberley Fielding is a nutrition coach, chef, and mother of three college students. She has a Bachelors degree in Biology from Cal Poly, San Luis Obispo, and has continued her education with nursing and nutrition classes.

Index